ADVANCES IN

Anesthesia

**Editor-in-Chief
Thomas M. McLoughlin, MD**

ELSEVIER

An Imprint of Elsevier, Inc.

PHILADELPHIA   LONDON   TORONTO   MONTREAL   SYDNEY   TOKYO

Vice President, Continuity Publishing: Kimberly Murphy
Editor: Yonah Korngold

Reprints: For copies of 100 or more of articles in this publication, please contact the Commercial Reprints Department, Elsevier Inc., 360 Park Avenue South, New York, NY 10010-1710. Tel: (212) 633-3812; Fax: (212) 462-1935; E-mail: reprints@elsevier.com.

Editorial Office:
Elsevier
1600 John F. Kennedy Blvd,
Suite 1800
Philadelphia, PA 19103-2899

International Standard Serial Number: 0737-6146
International Standard Book Number-13: 978-0-323-08404-8

Printed and bound by CPI Group (UK) Ltd, Croydon, CR0 4YY
Transferred to Digital Print 2011

ADVANCES IN
Anesthesia

Editor-in-Chief

THOMAS M. MCLOUGHLIN, MD, Associate Chief Medical Officer, Chair, Department of Anesthesiology, Lehigh Valley Health Network, Allentown, PA; and Professor of Surgery, Division of Surgical Anesthesiology, University of South Florida College of Medicine, Tampa, Florida

Associate Editors

JOEL O. JOHNSON, MD, PhD, Professor, Department of Anesthesiology, University of Wisconsin, Madison, Wisconsin

FRANCIS V. SALINAS, MD, Deputy Chief of Anesthesia; Section Head of Orthopedic Anesthesia; and Coordinator of Ultrasound-Guided Regional Anesthesia Education, Virginia Mason Medical Center Department of Anesthesiology, Seattle, Washington

CONTRIBUTORS

JAMES E. CALDWELL, MB, ChB, Professor, Department of Anesthesia and Perioperative Medicine, University of California, San Francisco, California

CHRISTOPHER M. DUNCAN, MD, Instructor of Anesthesiology, Department of Anesthesiology, Mayo Clinic College of Medicine, Rochester, Minnesota

DANIEL A. EMMERT, MD, PhD, Fellow, Cardiothoracic Anesthesiology, Department of Anesthesiology, Washington University in St Louis School of Medicine, St Louis, Missouri

JAMES R. HEBL, MD, Associate Professor of Anesthesiology, Department of Anesthesiology, Mayo Clinic College of Medicine, Rochester, Minnesota

ADAM K. JACOB, MD, Assistant Professor of Anesthesiology, Department of Anesthesiology, Mayo Clinic College of Medicine, Rochester, Minnesota

REBECCA L. JOHNSON, MD, Regional Anesthesia Fellow, Department of Anesthesiology, Mayo Clinic College of Medicine, Rochester, Minnesota

SANDRA L. KOPP, MD, Assistant Professor of Anesthesiology, Department of Anesthesiology, Mayo Clinic College of Medicine, Rochester, Minnesota

ISAAC LYNCH, MD, Instructor, Critical Care and Trauma Anesthesiology, Department of Anesthesiology, Washington University in St Louis School of Medicine, St Louis, Missouri

CARI L. MEYER, MD, Department of Anesthesiology, University of Wisconsin School of Medicine and Public Health, Madison, Wisconsin

CARRIE A. SCHROEDER, DVM, Diplomate, American College of Veterinary Anaesthesia; Adjunct Clinical Instructor in Anesthesiology, Department of Surgical Sciences, School of Veterinary Medicine, University of Wisconsin, Madison, Wisconsin

LESLEY J. SMITH, DVM, Diplomate, American College of Veterinary Anaesthesia; Clinical Professor of Anesthesiology and Section Head, Department of Surgical Sciences, School of Veterinary Medicine, University of Wisconsin, Madison, Wisconsin

JOHN E. TETZLAFF, MD, Professor of Anesthesiology, Staff Anesthesiologist, Department of General Anesthesia, Anesthesiology Institute, Cleveland Clinic, Cleveland Clinic Lerner College of Medicine of Case Western Reserve University, Cleveland, Ohio

KHA M. TRAN, MD, Assistant Professor of Clinical Anesthesiology and Critical Care Medicine, Attending Anesthesiologist, Director, Fetal Anesthesia Team, Department of Anesthesia, Children's Hospital of Philadelphia, University of Pennsylvania School of Medicine, Philadelphia, Pennsylvania

MICHAEL H. WALL, MD, FCCM, Professor, Anesthesiology and Cardiothoracic Surgery, Department of Anesthesiology, Washington University in St Louis School of Medicine, St Louis, Missouri

ADVANCES IN
Anesthesia

CONTENTS

Occupational Hazards for the Pregnant Anesthesia Provider
Cari L. Meyer

Veterinary Anesthesia
Carrie A. Schroeder and Lesley J. Smith

Perioperative Considerations and Management in Patients with Intravascular Stents
Isaac Lynch, Daniel A. Emmert, and Michael H. Wall

Drug Diversion, Chemical Dependence, and Anesthesiology
John E. Tetzlaff

Anesthesia for Intrauterine Fetal Therapy and Ex Utero Intrapartum Therapy
Kha M. Tran

Clinical Pathways for Total Joint Arthroplasty: Essential Components for Success
Rebecca L. Johnson, Christopher M. Duncan, and James R. Hebl

Advances in Anesthesia 29 (2011) 1–18

ADVANCES IN ANESTHESIA

ELSEVIER
MOSBY

Regional Anesthesia in the Patient with Preexisting Neurologic Disorders

Adam K. Jacob, MD, Sandra L. Kopp, MD*

Department of Anesthesiology, Mayo Clinic College of Medicine, 200 First Street Southwest, Rochester, MN 55905, USA

The benefits of regional anesthesia have been repeatedly shown in numerous clinical studies for a wide spectrum of surgical procedures. In all cases, the benefits of a regional technique must be balanced against the potential risk for complications. One of the most debilitating complications is the development of a new or worsened neurologic deficit [1,2]. Numerous risk factors may influence the development of perioperative nerve injury [3]. Therefore, it is important that anesthesia providers are aware of these risk factors when selecting suitable candidates for a regional technique.

Patients with preexisting neurologic disorders present a unique challenge to the anesthesiologist who is contemplating a regional anesthetic technique (neuraxial or peripheral nerve block) because the presence of preexisting deficits signifies neural compromise. Historically, the most conservative approach was to avoid regional anesthesia in patients with preexisting neurologic disorders to avoid further nerve injury. However, the decision to proceed with regional anesthesia should be made on a case-by-case basis because selected patients may benefit from a regional anesthetic technique compared with other anesthetic or analgesic options. If a regional technique is considered, a complete preoperative assessment of the patient's baseline neurologic status is critical and impossible to reproduce after an injury occurs.

This article discusses the mechanism of neurologic injury in the perioperative period, the pathophysiology of several central and peripheral neuromuscular disorders, and the role of regional anesthesia in the management of patients with these preexisting neurologic conditions.

THE DOUBLE-CRUSH PHENOMENON

A concern of anesthesiologists caring for patients with preexisting neurologic disease is the potential that the underlying neurologic condition may worsen or a new neurologic deficit may develop during the perioperative period. It

The authors have nothing to disclose.

*Corresponding author. E-mail address: kopp.sandra@mayo.edu

0737-6146/11/$ – see front matter
doi:10.1016/j.aan.2011.07.001

has been suggested that the presence of preexisting clinical or subclinical neural compromise may increase the risk for new or worsened perioperative nerve injury [3]. The double-crush phenomenon refers to the coexistence of at least 2 injurious insults or lesions along the course of a nerve. Upton and McComas [4] first described the double-crush syndrome in 1973, suggesting that a nerve with preexisting neural compromise was more susceptible to damage at another site (Fig. 1). Furthermore, the second site of injury may occur at any point along the pathway of neural transmission [5]. Although originally postulated to result from serial compressions or constraints in axonal flow, the concept of double-crush has been extrapolated to include other conditions such as inherited neurologic disorders or exposure to a metabolic, toxic, traumatic, or ischemic insult that serves as either the primary or secondary neural compromise.

Several patient-related and procedure-related characteristics have been associated with an increased risk for developing a new or worsened perioperative neurologic deficit. In general, patients with preexisting neurologic disorders

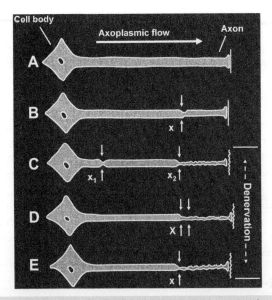

Fig. 1. Various types of neural lesions resulting in denervation. Amount of axoplasmic flow is indicated by the degree of shading. Complete loss of axoplasmic material results in denervation (C–E). (A) Normal, healthy neuron. (B) Neuron with mild compression at a single site (x) is insufficient to result in denervation distal to the injury. (C) Neuron with mild compression at 2 separate sites (x_1 and x_2) results in denervation distal to x_2. (D) Neuron with severe compression at a single location (x) results in denervation distal to x. (E) Neuron with preexisting clinical or subclinical disease (metabolic, toxic, ischemic) and compression at single site (x) resulting in denervation distal to x. (*Reproduced from* Hebl J. Peripheral nerve injury. In: Neal JM, Rathmell JP, editors. Complications in regional anesthesia and pain medicine. 1st edition. Saunders; 2006. p. 125–40; with permission.)

are assumed to have 1 risk factor (ie, the first crush) for new or worsened peri-operative nerve injury caused by their intrinsic disease. The so-called second crush may result from surgical-related risk factors such as intraoperative trauma or stretch, vascular compromise, hematoma formation, tourniquet ischemia, or constrictive dressings or regional anesthetic-related risk factors like mechanical trauma secondary to needle or catheter placement, ischemic injury caused by epinephrine additive, or chemical injury from local anesthetic neurotoxicity [3].

PERIPHERAL NERVOUS SYSTEM DISORDERS

The peripheral nervous system is composed of numerous cell types and elements that serve diverse motor, sensory, and autonomic functions. Signs and symptoms of impaired function depend on the severity and distribution of a nerve injury as well as the neural elements affected. More than 100 types of peripheral neuropathy have been identified, each with its own characteristic set of symptoms, pattern of development, and prognosis. Peripheral nerve disorders are commonly divided into hereditary and acquired forms.

Hereditary peripheral neuropathy

Inherited neuropathies represent a complex, heterogeneous group of diseases that often share the features of insidious onset and indolent course in periods of years to decades. A wide range of genotypes may result in phenotypes ranging from mild symptoms and subclinical disease, to severe, debilitating conditions. The most common inherited neuropathies are a group of disorders collectively referred to as Charcot-Marie-Tooth disease (CMTD), which affects approximately 1 in 2500 people, often beginning during childhood [6]. With multiple subtypes, CMTD neuropathies result from mutations in more than 30 genes responsible for manufacturing neurons or the myelin sheath [7]. Hallmarks of typical CMTD include extreme weakening and wasting of muscles in the lower legs and feet, gait abnormalities, loss of tendon reflexes, and numbness in the lower limbs.

The reported use of peripheral [8,9] or central [10–13] regional anesthetic techniques in patients with CMTD has been limited to case series and reports. All patients made uneventful recoveries without worsening of their neurologic conditions. Two cases involving single-injection technique (epidural anesthesia using 18 mL 0.75% ropivacaine [11], supraclavicular analgesia using 30 mL 0.5% bupivacaine [8]) reported a prolonged effect (12 hours and 30 hours, respectively) of the regional technique compared with the anticipated duration. In both cases, the use of higher concentration local anesthetic may have played a role in delayed recovery.

Hereditary neuropathy with liability to pressure palsy (HNPP) is another rare, inherited, demyelinating neuropathy in which individuals suffer from repeated motor and sensory neuropathies (pressure palsies) following brief nerve compression or mild trauma. Discovered in the early 1990s, HNPP has been linked to a mutation on the PMP-22 gene resulting in reduced myelin production. Evidence discussing the use of any regional technique in the setting of HNPP has been limited to a single case report. Lepske and Alderson [14] reported the successful use of labor epidural analgesia in a 24-year-old parturient with HNPP. The patient made an uneventful recovery without worsening of her neurologic condition.

Although we are unable to draw any formal conclusions about safety and use of regional anesthesia in patients with inherited peripheral neuropathies, case reports suggest that peripheral and central regional techniques may be used without worsening a patient's neurologic condition. However, caution should be used to minimize all other patient, surgical, and anesthetic risk factors for perioperative nerve injury when considering use of a regional technique.

Acquired peripheral neuropathy

Based on the double-crush phenomenon, it has been suggested that patients with a history of chronic neural compromise secondary to ischemic (peripheral vascular disease or microangiopathy), metabolic (diabetes mellitus) or toxic (chemotherapy) conditions may be at an increased risk of worsening neurologic injury following neuraxial or peripheral nerve blockade [15–18]. Diabetes mellitus is the most common cause of systemic polyneuropathy. The frequency of diabetic polyneuropathy ranges from 4% to 8% at the time of disease presentation to 50% of patients with chronic disease. Although many patients may be asymptomatic, nearly all have evidence of abnormal nerve conduction [19,20].

The pathophysiology of diabetic polyneuropathy seems to be multifactorial and is not well understood. Axonal degeneration can occur following disrupted delivery of essential nutritives (oxygen, blood, adenosine triphosphate, glucose) to the axon. There is concern that local anesthetics used for peripheral nerve blockade are more neurotoxic in the patient with diabetes mellitus [21–23]. Furthermore, the use of epinephrine additive may further reduce neural blood flow, leading to functional and/or structural changes [24]. Based on animal data, Kalichman and Calcutt [17] hypothesized that diabetic nerve fibers may be more susceptible to local anesthetic neurotoxicity for 2 reasons: (1) the nerves are already compromised because of chronic ischemic hypoxia; and (2) the nerves are exposed to larger concentrations of local anesthetics because of decreased blood flow. Kroin and colleagues [25] showed that the duration of sciatic nerve blockade in streptozotocin-induced diabetic rats was prolonged compared with nondiabetic rats. This finding has been supported clinically with data that suggest that the success rate of peripheral nerve blockade is higher in adult diabetic patients compared with nondiabetic patients [26]. However, there are few data to quantify the potential risk of peripheral nerve blockade in the diabetic patient. Further investigations are required to determine the incidence of neurologic complications following peripheral nerve blockade in diabetic patients as well the usefulness of modifications in local anesthetic dosing or nerve block technique.

A recent retrospective review evaluated neurologic complications in patients with preexisting peripheral sensorimotor neuropathy or diabetic polyneuropathy who subsequently underwent neuraxial anesthesia or analgesia [27]. Of the 567 patients studied, 2 (0.4%; 95% confidence interval [CI] 0.1%–1.3%) experienced new or progressive postoperative neurologic deficits compared with preoperative findings. The investigators determined that, although the risk of severe postoperative neurologic injury in this population is rare, it seems to be higher than that reported for the general population [28]. Although the role of the neuraxial blockade in the postoperative findings was unclear, it may have been a contributing factor in patients with already vulnerable nerves.

Another category of acquired peripheral neuropathy with increasing awareness among clinicians is inflammatory neuropathy. One of the most common forms of inflammatory neuropathy is Guillain-Barré syndrome (GBS). Also known as acute inflammatory polyneuropathy or acute inflammatory demyelinating polyneuropathy, GBS is an immune-mediated demyelinating condition evoked by antecedent respiratory or gastrointestinal infection that results in rapidly progressive sensory and motor changes. New cases of GBS have been reported after surgical or obstetric procedures with or without regional anesthesia [29–38]. Cases of GBS that have developed after epidural and spinal anesthesia [29,33,35,39] have led some investigators to propose that exposure to the medications commonly used in neuraxial techniques (eg, bupivacaine) may serve as another antecedent immune-mediated cause for GBS [35]. However, modern theories of GBS cause do not acknowledge this association [40].

There are no specific guidelines regarding anesthetic management of patients with GBS. Several investigators have reported cases in which a neuraxial technique was used in parturients with GBS for labor analgesia or cesarean delivery [36,41–45]. Although most cases reported that patients' neurologic condition was unchanged after the resolution of the regional anesthetic [41–45], 1 patient's neurologic status significantly worsened after patient-controlled epidural labor analgesia with 0.2% ropivacaine and sufentanil (1 μg/mL) [36]. This patient developed progressive lower extremity weakness that persisted for greater than 4 months after delivery but also concurrently developed facial and upper extremity weakness. Therefore, it is unclear whether the neuraxial technique directly contributed to the patients decline, or whether the patient's symptoms progressed because of the natural course of the disease.

As with inherited peripheral neuropathies, it is not possible to make conclusions about safety and use of regional anesthesia in patients with acquired peripheral neuropathy. Patients with clinical or subclinical diabetic neuropathy seem to be at higher risk for neurologic complications after regional anesthesia compared with the general public, but the risk remains small and each case must be individually considered to determine whether the benefit outweighs the potential risk. Regarding GBS, the overall incidence is extremely low and case reports suggest that central regional techniques may be used without worsening a patient's neurologic condition. No evidence exists regarding the role of peripheral nerve blockade and patients with GBS. Therefore, caution must be used when considering the potential risk for complications after a regional technique compared with other anesthetic techniques [46].

CENTRAL NERVOUS SYSTEM DISORDERS

Patients with preexisting disorders of the central nervous system have historically not been offered a neuraxial anesthetic technique because of a fear of worsening the neurologic outcome [47–50]. One of the most common disorders of the central nervous system is multiple sclerosis. Multiple sclerosis is a chronic, degenerative disease of the central nervous system characterized by focal demyelination in the spinal cord and brain. The demyelination process causes a fluctuating conduction block that results in the waxing and waning that is characteristic of the disease. Signs and symptoms include sensory or motor deficits, diplopia or vision loss, bowel or bladder dysfunction, and ataxia.

Several factors common to surgery can negatively affect the disease process, including hyperpyrexia, emotional stress, and infection [51]. The mechanism of worsening neurologic function in patients with multiple sclerosis is unclear and may occur coincidentally in the postoperative period independently of the anesthetic technique. The lack of myelin may leave the spinal cord more susceptible to the neurotoxic effects of local anesthetics [52]. Epidural anesthesia has been recommended rather than spinal anesthesia because the concentration of local anesthetic in the white matter of the spinal cord is one-fourth the level after epidural injection [52]. A recent report of severe brachial plexopathy following an interscalene nerve block in a patient with multiple sclerosis caused concern regarding the performance of peripheral nerve blockade in this patient population [53]. Historically, it was believed that multiple sclerosis was solely a disease of the central nervous system, although data exist suggesting that peripheral nervous system involvement may also occur [54,55].

The recommendation by Dripps and Vandam [50] in 1956 to avoid neuraxial blockade in patients with preexisting neurologic disorders has influenced clinical management for the last several decades. Several theoretic mechanisms have been proposed based on the double-crush phenomenon, including neurologic injury from needle-induced or catheter-induced trauma, local anesthetic neurotoxicity, and neural ischemia caused by local anesthetic additives. The avoidance of neuraxial techniques in this patient population may also be caused by physician and patient biases or potential medicolegal concerns. Several confounding factors such as age, body habitus, surgical trauma, tourniquet times and pressures, positioning, and anesthetic technique make determining the cause of worsening neurologic deficits difficult.

A recent review identified 139 patients in a 12-year period who had a history of a central nervous system disorder and subsequently underwent neuraxial anesthesia [48]. The preoperative neurologic disorders included primarily multiple sclerosis, postpolio syndrome, amyotrophic lateral sclerosis, and traumatic spinal cord injury. In contrast with the findings by Dripps and Vandam [50] decades ago, the investigators concluded that, compared with the preoperative deficits, no new or worsening postoperative neurologic deficits were identified (0.0%; 95% CI, 0.0%–0.3%), despite 74% of the patients reporting active neurologic symptoms or deficits (paresthesias, dysesthesias, hyperreflexia, or sensorimotor deficits) in the immediate preoperative period and subsequently received standard doses of local anesthetics. Although this is currently the largest case series, 2 smaller reviews in parturients receiving small doses of local anesthetics for labor analgesia have reported similar results [56,57].

Further investigations with a larger number of patients are needed to make definitive recommendations, although the current data suggest that the decision to perform neuraxial anesthesia in patients with preexisting central nervous system disorders should be based on the risks and benefits for each individual patient. Recent investigations suggest that the risks previously associated with neuraxial blockade in patients with central nervous system disorders may be less frequent than was previously believed.

SPINAL STENOSIS AND LUMBAR DISK DISEASE

Spinal stenosis is caused by age-related changes in the disks and facet joints of the spine that ultimately lead to narrowing of the spinal canal or neural foramina. These age-related changes include disk degeneration, facet joint hypertrophy, osteophyte formation, and infolding of the ligamentum flavum. The exact mechanism by which spinal nerve root compression results in signs or symptoms of spinal stenosis (back/leg radicular pain, worsening with extension and alleviated with flexion) is not completely understood [58]. Preexisting spinal stenosis or lumbar disk disease has been proposed as a risk factor for complications following a neuraxial (spinal or epidural) technique. The proposed mechanisms of injury include mechanical trauma [59,60], local anesthetic neurotoxicity [61,62], ischemia [63–65], or a multifactorial cause [66,67]. Pathophysiologically, patients with spinal stenosis have less room available for collections of fluid (blood or local anesthetic) around the neuraxis without a concomitant increase in pressure. It has been speculated that this competition for central canal space may partially explain why symptomatic epidural hematomas are more common in elderly patients [61].

Two recent case series and several case reports suggest that undiagnosed spinal stenosis may be a significant risk factor for neurologic complications following neuraxial blockade [59,61,63,66,68]. Hebl and colleagues [66] performed a retrospective review of patients with preexisting spinal stenosis or lumbar disk disease with and without a history of prior spinal surgery and concluded that these patients are at an increased risk for the development or worsening of neurologic deficits compared with the general population undergoing a neuraxial technique. In addition, patients with a history of multiple neurologic disorders, including spinal stenosis, radiculopathy, or peripheral neuropathy, seemed to have an even higher risk of injury. A large epidemiologic study in Sweden revealed similar trends [61]. During the 10-year study period, approximately 1,260,000 spinal and 450,000 epidural blocks were reviewed with a total of 127 serious complications identified, including 85 patients with permanent neurologic injuries. Although 14 patients had preexisting spinal stenosis, 13 of these were diagnosed during the workup of the neurologic injury in the postoperative period. The investigators concluded that the incidence of severe anesthesia-related complications may not be as low as was previously reported, and preexisting spinal canal disorders may be a neglected risk factor.

Although it seems that patients with spinal stenosis may have an increased incidence of neurologic complications following neuraxial block, the existing literature lacks a comparison of surgical patients with similar spinal disorders undergoing general anesthesia. Therefore, it is unclear whether the neurologic complications are caused by surgical factors, the anesthetic technique, natural progression of the spinal disorder, or a combination of these factors.

MYOPATHIC DISORDERS

The myopathies are neuromuscular disorders in which the primary symptom is muscle weakness caused by dysfunction of muscle fiber. Myopathies can be inherited (eg, muscular dystrophy) or acquired (eg, polymyositis). As a whole, patients with myopathic conditions are at increased risk for perioperative cardiac and pulmonary complications, temperature dysregulation, rhabdomyolysis, and autonomic lability following general anesthesia [69]. Therefore, avoidance of neuromuscular blocking medications and inhaled anesthetics may be an attractive option if the procedure is suitable for a regional technique.

Duchenne muscular dystrophy (DMD) and Becker muscular dystrophy (BMD) are caused by mutations of the dystrophin gene resulting in muscle fiber degeneration and weakness. Both are inherited as X-linked recessive traits and have varying clinical characteristics. DMD is associated with the most severe clinical symptoms presenting early in life, whereas BMD has a similar presentation but presents later and has a milder clinical course. Although many procedures (eg, scoliosis correction) may not be suitable for regional anesthesia, case reports [70–72] have described the safe use of spinal and epidural anesthesia in patients with muscular dystrophy or symptomatic carriers of muscular dystrophy without worsening the patients' neuromuscular condition.

The myotonic dystrophies (DM) are inherited multisystem disorders characterized by progressive weakness, myotonia, cataracts, endocrine disturbances, and functional abnormalities of the cardiorespiratory and gastrointestinal systems. The 2 main forms of myotonic dystrophy, DM1 (Steinert disease) and DM2, are similar in that both are multisystem disorders. However, DM2 is generally less severe than DM1. A recent case series [73] and retrospective observational study [74] described the safe use of spinal, epidural, and peripheral regional anesthesia in a combined total of 38 patients with DM2. Fewer patients receiving regional or local anesthesia experienced worsening of their neurologic condition in the perioperative period compared with patients who underwent general anesthesia [74].

Patients with myopathic disorders are at increased risk for perioperative complications, regardless of anesthetic technique. Limited evidence suggests that regional techniques may be used safely on these patients in certain circumstances, but the existing literature is insufficient to clearly show safety or superiority of regional anesthesia compared with general anesthesia in patients with myopathies.

INTRACRANIAL TUMORS, ANEURYSMS, AND ARTERIOVENOUS MALFORMATIONS

Patients with intracranial masses (primary or metastatic brain tumors) and vascular lesions (aneurysms or arteriovenous malformations) are at an increased risk of neurologic compromise during neuraxial anesthesia. Dural puncture is contraindicated in patients with increased intracranial pressure because the acute leakage of cerebrospinal fluid (CSF) caused by dural puncture leads to decreased CSF pressure and may cause cerebellar herniation [75]. In patients with uncorrected vascular malformations, the decreased CSF pressure may increase the aneurysmal transmural pressure gradient and ultimately result in hemorrhage. Epidural and caudal anesthesia are similarly contraindicated in this patient population because of the risk of unintended dural puncture as well as the risk of increasing the intracranial pressure following injection of local anesthetic into the epidural space. Wedel and Mulroy [76] reported a case of hemiparesis caused by occult arteriovenous malformation rupture following an inadvertent dural puncture during epidural placement.

SEIZURE DISORDERS AND EPILEPSY

Seizure is defined as the clinical manifestation of abnormally hyperexcitable cortical neurons. Although all patients with epilepsy have seizures, many patients have a single seizure during life and are not considered to have epilepsy. A population-based epidemiologic study from Rochester (MN) found that the cumulative incidence of epilepsy to age 74 years is 3.0%, with an incidence of any convulsive disorder approaching 10% [77]. Therefore, it is common for a patient with the diagnosis of a seizure disorder to present for a surgical procedure in which regional anesthesia or analgesia may be considered.

Local anesthetic systemic toxicity is a potential risk for all patients undergoing regional anesthesia, particularly during procedures that require a large dose of local anesthetic (eg, caudal or epidural). Systemic local anesthetic toxicity presents as a spectrum of neurologic signs and symptoms that worsen as plasma drug levels continue to increase. At low blood levels, local anesthetics decrease cerebral blood flow, metabolism, and electrical activity, and are potent anticonvulsants. Conversely, at higher levels, they act as proconvulsants by lowering the seizure threshold within the cerebral cortex, amygdala, and hippocampus, usually leading to a generalized convulsion [78]. As the serum drug level continues to increase, both inhibitory and excitatory neural pathways are blocked, resulting in generalized central nervous system depression.

Common factors that may provoke seizure activity in patients with a history of a seizure disorder include fluctuations in antiepileptic drug blood levels, sleep deprivation, fatigue, stress, excessive alcohol intake, and menstruation [79,80]. A recent review of patients with a history of a seizure disorder that underwent regional anesthesia requiring large doses of local anesthetic concluded that most seizures occurring in the perioperative period were likely related to the patient's underlying condition and that regional anesthesia in these patients is not contraindicated [81]. In addition, the likelihood of a postoperative seizure is increased in patients with a recent seizure; therefore it is essential to be prepared to treat seizure activity, regardless of the anesthetic technique [81,82].

POSTSURGICAL INFLAMMATORY NEUROPATHY

Recently anesthesiologists have become aware that an autoimmune or inflammatory process may be the cause of severe postoperative neurologic deficits [83]. Staff and colleagues [84] recently described a series of 33 patients who developed postsurgical inflammatory neuropathy within 30 days of surgery. The diagnosis was confirmed in most patients following a nerve biopsy. Postsurgical inflammatory neuropathy is believed to be an idiopathic, immune-mediated response to a physiologic stress such as infection, a vaccination, or a surgical procedure [84]. The neuropathy may present with focal, multifocal, or diffuse neurologic deficits in the setting of negative radiologic imaging. Complicating the diagnosis, the onset of neurologic deficits may not be apparent in the immediate postoperative period and the deficits may be in an anatomic distribution remote from the surgical site or regional anesthetic technique. Risk factors or potential triggers for postsurgical inflammatory neuropathy include malignancy, diabetes mellitus, tobacco use, systemic infection, volatile anesthetic use, and recent blood transfusion [84]. Suppression of the immune response with prolonged, high-dose corticosteroids or intravenous immunoglobulin is the current treatment of choice. The goal of treatment is to blunt the inflammatory response and allow for axonal regeneration. Most patients improve with the current treatment, with the sensory deficits and pain improving before the motor deficits [84].

The role of inflammatory mechanisms in postoperative neuropathies is unappreciated and not well characterized, specifically within the anesthesiology literature. As a result, anesthesia providers and surgeons rarely consider this potential cause of nerve injury when evaluating patients with postoperative deficits. This omission is problematic, because the usual approach of watchful waiting and conservative management is not effective in patients with postsurgical inflammatory neuropathy. Instead, this is a clinical condition that must be suspected and identified (nerve biopsy) early in the disease process so that aggressive immunotherapy can be initiated [84].

EVALUATION OF NEW OR WORSENED NEUROLOGIC DEFICIT

Despite meticulous regional anesthesia technique, neurologic complications occur. However, neurologic complications are rare and usually resolve within days to weeks. Because of the infrequent occurrence of a significant nerve injury, many anesthesiologists are unfamiliar with the diagnosis and management of such an injury. This unfamiliarity may lead to a delay in the diagnosis and treatment, potentially worsening the outcome. In the early postoperative period, as many as 15% of patients undergoing peripheral nerve blockade may experience a mild paresthesia [85]. Most of these symptoms resolve in a period of days to weeks and require no formal evaluation. The greatest challenge is to identify patients who have experienced a significant perioperative nerve injury and facilitate a proper evaluation.

Seddon [86] proposed the first system to classify nerve injuries in 1942 using 3 terms (neurapraxia, axonotmesis, neurotmesis) to describe increasingly severe degrees of neural injury. In 1951, Sunderland [87] proposed an alternative classification system for peripheral nerve injuries with greater clinical usefulness and relevance than the Seddon system. A modified summary of the Sunderland Classification System is presented in Table 1.

Mild nerve injury

With a mild injury, the clinical deficit is primarily caused by a block in the conduction of nerve impulses through the affected nerve segment (neurapraxia). Recovery typically occurs in days to weeks if the cause has been removed and the damage is not severe enough to cause structural changes in the myelin sheath [88]. Patients without objective evidence of neural deficits can be reassured that a complete recovery is expected. However, if symptoms do not improve in a period of 2 to 3 weeks, or if the symptoms worsen at any time, a neurologic consultation should be requested [3].

Severe nerve injury

Severe nerve injuries lead to axonal degeneration caused by axonotmesis. Recovery depends on axonal regeneration and is often delayed and incomplete. Patients with evidence of moderate to severe deficits should be referred for an early neurologic consultation. After a thorough history and examination, the neurologist will direct the appropriate imaging and/or neurophysiologic testing. The prognosis largely depends on the integrity of the remaining support structure in the nerve (epineurium and perineurium) [88].

Complete or progressive nerve injury

In the most severe injuries, the epineurium is disrupted (neurotmesis) and recovery is only possible following surgical repair. Patients complaining of severe or worsening symptoms should be referred for an urgent neurology workup. After a thorough history and physical examination, the patient will likely undergo imaging as well as neurophysiologic testing to aid in diagnosis and treatment.

A thorough history and physical examination is the first step in the diagnosis of a suspected peripheral nerve injury to establish baseline neurologic status. In addition to identifying and documenting the patient's signs and symptoms, it is important to review the surgical events that may contribute to postoperative nerve injury. These events include intraoperative nerve trauma or stretch, vascular injury and bleeding complications, prolonged tourniquet times, and extensive traction because of a difficult exposure.

Table 1
Sunderland classification of nerve injury

Degree of injury	Axonal nerve conduction	Wallerian degeneration	Endoneurial tube integrity	Loss of function	Recover/time course
Type I	Focally interrupted at site of injury	No	Maintained	Variable; often motor > sensory	Complete restoration of function within days to weeks
Type II	Interrupted distally from site of injury	Yes	Maintained	Transient loss of motor, sensory, and sympathetic function	Regeneration and functional recovery common within weeks to months
Type III	Interrupted distally from site of injury	Yes	Disrupted, scarring of endoneurium	Prolonged motor, sensory, and sympathetic deficits	Partial regeneration possible; however, complete return of function does not occur
Type IV	Interrupted distally from site of injury	Yes	Disrupted, fascicle perineurium also disrupted	Severe loss of motor, sensory, and sympathetic function; cell-body mortality high	Deficits generally permanent; prognosis for significant return of function poor without surgery
Type V	Interrupted distally from site of injury	Yes	Disrupted, external epineurium severed	Severe loss of motor, sensory, and sympathetic function; cell-body mortality high	Possibility of significant return of function remote, even with surgery

Reproduced from Hebl J. Peripheral nerve injury. In: Neal JM, Rathmell JP, editors. Complications in regional anesthesia and pain medicine. 1st edition. Saunders; 2006. p. 125–40; with permission.

A complete neurologic examination by a neurologist or neurosurgeon should take place as soon as a postoperative nerve deficit is suspected. Neuraxial injuries should be suspected in patients with a motor block out of proportion to that expected from the regional technique, a motor block that is prolonged, or worsening of sensory or motor block that had shown signs of regression. Patients suspected of having a compressive lesion of the neuraxis require rapid evaluation and treatment because the prospect of recovery decreases if the time from symptoms to decompression exceeds 8 hours [89]. Magnetic resonance imaging (MRI) is the imaging modality of choice for identifying spinal canal disorders. However, if MRI is unavailable, computed tomography (CT) should be used to avoid delaying the evaluation.

ELECTROPHYSIOLOGIC TESTING

Electrophysiologic testing aids in defining the neurogenic basis of the deficit (axon loss or demyelination) and ultimately assists in localizing the site of the lesion. It may also guide prognosis by determining the severity of the injury. A limitation of electrophysiologic testing is its inability to discern the cause of the nerve injury [88]. For example, in a patient complaining of weakness and numbness in the foot following a total knee replacement, electrophysiologic testing may confirm the presence of a sciatic neuropathy and identify the site of injury at the level of the knee. It may also be able to determine whether the injury is acute or chronic, and may even provide information about the severity of the injury, but it cannot identify the cause. The cause needs to be inferred based on the clinical information provided, such as past medical history (diabetes, preexisting nerve injury, presence of a valgus deformity), the type of anesthetic used (neuraxial vs general), the use of peripheral nerve blocks and level of placement, and surgical factors including the use of a tourniquet.

Electromyography

Electromyography (EMG) involves inserting an electrode into a muscle to record the electrical activity. The motor unit consists of the anterior horn cell, the axon and neuromuscular junctions, and the muscle fibers it innervates. EMG is used to obtain information regarding the pathologic site of a disorder within the motor unit [88]. Although the patterns of affected muscles obtained using EMG may help localize a lesion to the spinal cord, nerve roots, plexuses, or peripheral nerves, EMG cannot provide a definitive cause of the injury. EMG can also provide information regarding the timing or onset of the injury as well as its chronicity. Many disease processes take weeks to evolve and are not apparent on EMG immediately after the injury. Despite this, a baseline EMG immediately after suspicion of nerve injury aids in ruling out a preexisting nerve injury or subclinical disorder that was previously undiagnosed.

Nerve conduction studies

Nerve conduction studies are used to evaluate the functional integrity of nerves and aid in localization of focal lesions. Nerve conduction studies can be used to assess the function of motor and sensory nerves. In motor studies, the nerve is stimulated at 2 or more points along its course, and the electrical response is recorded from one of the muscles it innervates. A reduction in the conduction velocity at one point, compared with stimulation at a more distal site, may indicate a conduction block, acute axon loss, or anomalous innervation [88]. Sensory conduction studies involve stimulating nerve fibers at one point and recording the nerve action potentials obtained at another site. The latency of the response and the sensory nerve action potential are a reflection of the number of functioning sensory axons [88]. The primary goals of a nerve conduction study are to assess the number of functioning axons (amplitude) as well as the state of the myelin (conduction velocity) within the axons.

TIMING OF EVALUATION
The optimal timing of electrophysiologic testing depends on the reasons for ordering such an evaluation. Occasionally, it is useful to have patients undergo evaluation within the first 2 to 3 days following an injury, especially in the setting of postoperative weakness or sensory changes. An early examination can confirm that there is a nerve lesion present, in addition to identifying an underlying, chronic deficit.

In time, the electrophysiology changes after a new nerve injury. Therefore, performing the evaluation approximately 4 weeks after an injury can provide more information regarding the nature, site, and severity of the lesion. Serial studies are often not required because progress is best monitored clinically.

SUMMARY
Patients with preexisting neurologic disorders present a unique challenge to the anesthesiologist who is contemplating a regional anesthetic technique. A thorough preoperative assessment is vital to establish the patient's baseline neurologic status. Anesthesia providers should be aware of the patient and procedural risk factors for postoperative neurologic complications during their selection of suitable candidates for a central or peripheral block, and adapt their technique to minimize these risks as much as possible. Although a preexisting neurologic disorder is not an absolute contraindication to regional anesthesia, the decision to proceed with a regional technique should be made on a case-by-case basis because select patients may benefit from a regional anesthetic technique compared with other anesthetic or analgesic options.

References
[1] Warner MA, Martin JT, Schroeder DR, et al. Lower-extremity motor neuropathy associated with surgery performed on patients in a lithotomy position. Anesthesiology 1994;81(1): 6–12.
[2] Warner MA, Warner ME, Martin JT. Ulnar neuropathy. Incidence, outcome, and risk factors in sedated or anesthetized patients. Anesthesiology 1994;81(6):1332–40.
[3] Neal JM, Bernards CM, Hadzic A, et al. ASRA practice advisory on neurologic complications in regional anesthesia and pain medicine. Reg Anesth Pain Med 2008;33(5):404–15.

[4] Upton AR, McComas AJ. The double crush in nerve entrapment syndromes. Lancet 1973;2(7825):359–62.

[5] Osterman AL. The double crush syndrome. Orthop Clin North Am 1988;19(1):147–55.

[6] Skre H. Genetic and clinical aspects of Charcot-Marie-Tooth's disease. Clin Genet 1974;6(2):98–118.

[7] Saporta AS, Sottile SL, Miller LJ, et al. Charcot-Marie-Tooth disease subtypes and genetic testing strategies. Ann Neurol 2011;69(1):22–33.

[8] Bui AH, Marco AP. Peripheral nerve blockade in a patient with Charcot-Marie-Tooth disease. Can J Anaesth 2008;55(10):718–9.

[9] Dhir S, Balasubramanian S, Ross D. Ultrasound-guided peripheral regional blockade in patients with Charcot-Marie-Tooth disease: a review of three cases. Can J Anaesth 2008;55(8):515–20.

[10] Fernandez Perez AB, Quesada Garcia C, Rodriguez Gonzalez O, et al. Obstetric epidural analgesia, a safe choice in a patient with Charcot-Marie-Tooth disease. Rev Esp Anestesiol Reanim 2011;58(4):255–6 [in Spanish].

[11] Schmitt HJ, Muenster T, Schmidt J. Central neural blockade in Charcot-Marie-Tooth disease. Can J Anaesth 2004;51(10):1049–50.

[12] Sugai K, Sugai Y. Epidural anesthesia for a patient with Charcot-Marie-Tooth disease, bronchial asthma and hypothyroidism. Masui 1989;38(5):688–91 [in Japanese].

[13] Tanaka S, Tsuchida H, Namiki A. Epidural anesthesia for a patient with Charcot-Marie-Tooth disease, mitral valve prolapse syndrome and IInd degree AV block. Masui 1994;43(6): 931–3 [in Japanese].

[14] Lepski GR, Alderson JD. Epidural analgesia in labour for a patient with hereditary neuropathy with liability to pressure palsy. Int J Obstet Anesth 2001;10(3):198–201.

[15] Hebl JR, Horlocker TT, Sorenson EJ, et al. Regional anesthesia does not increase the risk of postoperative neuropathy in patients undergoing ulnar nerve transposition. Anesth Analg 2001;93(6):1606–11, table of contents.

[16] Horlocker TT, O'Driscoll SW, Dinapoli RP. Recurring brachial plexus neuropathy in a diabetic patient after shoulder surgery and continuous interscalene block. Anesth Analg 2000;91(3):688–90.

[17] Kalichman MW, Calcutt NA. Local anesthetic-induced conduction block and nerve fiber injury in streptozotocin-diabetic rats. Anesthesiology 1992;77(5):941–7.

[18] Waters JH, Watson TB, Ward MG. Conus medullaris injury following both tetracaine and lidocaine spinal anesthesia. J Clin Anesth 1996;8(8):656–8.

[19] Dyck PJ, Kratz KM, Karnes JL, et al. The prevalence by staged severity of various types of diabetic neuropathy, retinopathy, and nephropathy in a population-based cohort: the Rochester Diabetic Neuropathy Study. Neurology 1993;43(4):817–24.

[20] Ross MA. Neuropathies associated with diabetes. Med Clin North Am 1993;77(1): 111–24.

[21] Neal JM. Effects of epinephrine in local anesthetics on the central and peripheral nervous systems: neurotoxicity and neural blood flow. Reg Anesth Pain Med 2003;28(2):124–34.

[22] Williams BA, Murinson BB. Diabetes mellitus and subclinical neuropathy: a call for new paths in peripheral nerve block research. Anesthesiology 2008;109(3):361–2.

[23] Williams BA, Murinson BB, Grable BR, et al. Future considerations for pharmacologic adjuvants in single-injection peripheral nerve blocks for patients with diabetes mellitus. Reg Anesth Pain Med 2009;34(5):445–57.

[24] Myers RR, Heckman HM. Effects of local anesthesia on nerve blood flow: studies using lidocaine with and without epinephrine. Anesthesiology 1989;71(5):757–62.

[25] Kroin JS, Buvanendran A, Williams DK, et al. Local anesthetic sciatic nerve block and nerve fiber damage in diabetic rats. Reg Anesth Pain Med 2010;35(4):343–50.

[26] Gebhard RE, Nielsen KC, Pietrobon R, et al. Diabetes mellitus, independent of body mass index, is associated with a "higher success" rate for supraclavicular brachial plexus blocks. Reg Anesth Pain Med 2009;34(5):404–7.

[27] Hebl JR, Kopp SL, Schroeder DR, et al. Neurologic complications after neuraxial anesthesia or analgesia in patients with preexisting peripheral sensorimotor neuropathy or diabetic polyneuropathy. Anesth Analg 2006;103(5):1294–9.

[28] Brull R, McCartney CJ, Chan VW, et al. Neurological complications after regional anesthesia: contemporary estimates of risk. Anesth Analg 2007;104(4):965–74.

[29] Gautier PE, Pierre PA, Van Obbergh LJ, et al. Guillain-Barre syndrome after obstetrical epidural analgesia. Reg Anesth 1989;14(5):251–2.

[30] Jones GD, Wilmshurst JM, Sykes K, et al. Guillain-Barre syndrome: delayed diagnosis following anaesthesia. Paediatr Anaesth 1999;9(6):539–42.

[31] Martin GG, Cueto OH, Acebal MR. Guillain-Barre syndrome following epidural anesthesia. Rev Esp Anestesiol Reanim 2008;55(5):323 [in Spanish].

[32] Olivier N, Laribi H, Pages M, et al. Recurrent Guillain-Barre syndrome after surgery. Rev Neurol (Paris) 2010;166(6–7):644–7 [in French].

[33] Rosenberg SK, Stacey BR. Postoperative Guillain-Barre syndrome, arachnoiditis, and epidural analgesia. Reg Anesth 1996;21(5):486–9.

[34] Shuert GT, Gamble JW. Guillain-Barre syndrome after mandibular surgery: report of case. J Oral Surg 1972;30(12):913–5.

[35] Steiner I, Argov Z, Cahan C, et al. Guillain-Barre syndrome after epidural anesthesia: direct nerve root damage may trigger disease. Neurology 1985;35(10):1473–5.

[36] Wiertlewski S, Magot A, Drapier S, et al. Worsening of neurologic symptoms after epidural anesthesia for labor in a Guillain-Barre patient. Anesth Analg 2004;98(3):825–7, table of contents.

[37] Rockel A, Wissel J, Rolfs A. Guillain-Barre syndrome in pregnancy—an indication for caesarian section? J Perinat Med 1994;22(5):393–8.

[38] Rolfs A, Bolik A. Guillain-Barre syndrome in pregnancy: reflections on immunopathogenesis. Acta Neurol Scand 1994;89(5):400–2.

[39] Flores-Barragan JM, Martinez-Palomeque G, Ibanez R, et al. Guillain-Barre syndrome as a complication of epidural anaesthesia. Rev Neurol 2006;42(10):631–2 [in Spanish].

[40] Hardy TA, Blum S, McCombe PA, et al. Guillain-Barre syndrome: modern theories of etiology. Curr Allergy Asthma Rep 2011;11(3):197–204.

[41] Brooks H, Christian AS, May AE. Pregnancy, anaesthesia and Guillain Barre syndrome. Anaesthesia 2000;55(9):894–8.

[42] Vassiliev DV, Nystrom EU, Leicht CH. Combined spinal and epidural anesthesia for labor and cesarean delivery in a patient with Guillain-Barre syndrome. Reg Anesth Pain Med 2001;26(2):174–6.

[43] Chan LY, Tsui MH, Leung TN. Guillain-Barre syndrome in pregnancy. Acta Obstet Gynecol Scand 2004;83(4):319–25.

[44] Alici HA, Cesur M, Erdem AF, et al. Repeated use of epidural anaesthesia for caesarean delivery in a patient with Guillain-Barre syndrome. Int J Obstet Anesth 2005;14(3):269–70.

[45] Kocabas S, Karaman S, Firat V, et al. Anesthetic management of Guillain-Barre syndrome in pregnancy. J Clin Anesth 2007;19(4):299–302.

[46] Feldman JM. Cardiac arrest after succinylcholine administration in a pregnant patient recovered from Guillain-Barre syndrome. Anesthesiology 1990;72(5):942–4.

[47] Bamford C, Sibley W, Laguna J. Anesthesia in multiple sclerosis. Can J Neurol Sci 1978;5(1):41–4.

[48] Hebl JR, Horlocker TT, Schroeder DR. Neuraxial anesthesia and analgesia in patients with preexisting central nervous system disorders. Anesth Analg 2006;103(1):223–8, table of contents.

[49] Keschner M. The effect of injuries and illness on the course of multiple sclerosis. Res Publ Assoc Res Nerv Ment Dis 1950;28:533–47.

[50] Dripps RD, Vandam LD. Exacerbation of pre-existing neurologic disease after spinal anesthesia. N Engl J Med 1956;255(18):843–9.

[51] Korn-Lubetzki I, Kahana E, Cooper G, et al. Activity of multiple sclerosis during pregnancy and puerperium. Ann Neurol 1984;16(2):229–31.

[52] Warren TM, Datta S, Ostheimer GW. Lumbar epidural anesthesia in a patient with multiple sclerosis. Anesth Analg 1982;61(12):1022–3.

[53] Koff MD, Cohen JA, McIntyre JJ, et al. Severe brachial plexopathy after an ultrasound-guided single-injection nerve block for total shoulder arthroplasty in a patient with multiple sclerosis. Anesthesiology 2008;108(2):325–8.

[54] Misawa S, Kuwabara S, Mori M, et al. Peripheral nerve demyelination in multiple sclerosis. Clin Neurophysiol 2008;119(8):1829–33.

[55] Sarova-Pinhas I, Achiron A, Gilad R, et al. Peripheral neuropathy in multiple sclerosis: a clinical and electrophysiologic study. Acta Neurol Scand 1995;91(4):234–8.

[56] Confavreux C, Hutchinson M, Hours MM, et al. Rate of pregnancy-related relapse in multiple sclerosis. Pregnancy in multiple sclerosis group. N Engl J Med 1998;339(5): 285–91.

[57] Crawford JS. Epidural analgesia for patients with chronic neurological disease. Anesth Analg 1983;62(6):621–2.

[58] Katz JN, Harris MB. Clinical practice. Lumbar spinal stenosis. N Engl J Med 2008;358(8): 818–25.

[59] Stambough JL, Stambough JB, Evans S. Acute cauda equina syndrome after total knee arthroplasty as a result of epidural anesthesia and spinal stenosis. J Arthroplasty 2000; 15(3):375–9.

[60] Tetzlaff JE, Dilger JA, Wu C, et al. Influence of lumbar spine pathology on the incidence of paresthesia during spinal anesthesia. Reg Anesth Pain Med 1998;23(6):560–3.

[61] Moen V, Dahlgren N, Irestedt L. Severe neurological complications after central neuraxial blockades in Sweden 1990-1999. Anesthesiology 2004;101(4):950–9.

[62] Yuen EC, Layzer RB, Weitz SR, et al. Neurologic complications of lumbar epidural anesthesia and analgesia. Neurology 1995;45(10):1795–801.

[63] de Seze MP, Sztark F, Janvier G, et al. Severe and long-lasting complications of the nerve root and spinal cord after central neuraxial blockade. Anesth Analg 2007;104(4):975–9.

[64] Hooten WM, Hogan MS, Sanemann TC, et al. Acute spinal pain during an attempted lumbar epidural blood patch in congenital lumbar spinal stenosis and epidural lipomatosis. Pain Physician 2008;11(1):87–90.

[65] Usubiaga JE, Wikinski JA, Usubiaga LE. Epidural pressure and its relation to spread of anesthetic solutions in epidural space. Anesth Analg 1967;46(4):440–6.

[66] Hebl JR, Horlocker TT, Kopp SL, et al. Neuraxial blockade in patients with preexisting spinal stenosis, lumbar disk disease, or prior spine surgery: efficacy and neurologic complications. Anesth Analg 2010;111(6):1511–9.

[67] Horlocker TT. Neuraxial blockade in patients with spinal stenosis: between a rock and a hard place. Anesth Analg 2010;110(1):13–5.

[68] Kubina P, Gupta A, Oscarsson A, et al. Two cases of cauda equina syndrome following spinal-epidural anesthesia. Reg Anesth 1997;22(5):447–50.

[69] Klingler W, Lehmann-Horn F, Jurkat-Rott K. Complications of anaesthesia in neuromuscular disorders. Neuromuscul Disord 2005;15(3):195–206.

[70] Caliskan E, Sener M, Kocum A, et al. Duchenne muscular dystrophy: how I do it? Regional or general anesthesia? Paediatr Anaesth 2009;19(6):624–5.

[71] Molyneux MK. Anaesthetic management during labour of a manifesting carrier of Duchenne muscular dystrophy. Int J Obstet Anesth 2005;14(1):58–61.

[72] Pash MP, Balaton J, Eagle C. Anaesthetic management of a parturient with severe muscular dystrophy, lumbar lordosis and a difficult airway. Can J Anaesth 1996;43(9):959–63.

[73] Weingarten TN, Hofer RE, Milone M, et al. Anesthesia and myotonic dystrophy type 2: a case series. Can J Anaesth 2010;57(3):248–55.

[74] Kirzinger L, Schmidt A, Kornblum C, et al. Side effects of anesthesia in DM2 as compared to DM1: a comparative retrospective study. Eur J Neurol 2010;17(6):842–5.

[75] Gower DJ, Baker AL, Bell WO, et al. Contraindications to lumbar puncture as defined by computed cranial tomography. J Neurol Neurosurg Psychiatry 1987;50(8):1071–4.

[76] Wedel DJ, Mulroy MF. Hemiparesis following dural puncture. Anesthesiology 1983;59(5): 475–7.

[77] Hauser WA, Annegers JF, Rocca WA. Descriptive epidemiology of epilepsy: contributions of population-based studies from Rochester, Minnesota. Mayo Clin Proc 1996;71(6): 576–86.

[78] DeToledo JC, Minagar A, Lowe MR. Lidocaine-induced seizures in patients with history of epilepsy: effect of antiepileptic drugs. Anesthesiology 2002;97(3):737–9.

[79] Paul F, Veauthier C, Fritz G, et al. Perioperative fluctuations of lamotrigine serum levels in patients undergoing epilepsy surgery. Seizure 2007;16(6):479–84.

[80] Sokic D, Ristic AJ, Vojvodic N, et al. Frequency, causes and phenomenology of late seizure recurrence in patients with juvenile myoclonic epilepsy after a long period of remission. Seizure 2007;16(6):533–7.

[81] Kopp SL, Wynd KP, Horlocker TT, et al. Regional blockade in patients with a history of a seizure disorder. Anesth Analg 2009;109(1):272–8.

[82] Niesen AD, Jacob AK, Aho LE, et al. Perioperative seizures in patients with a history of a seizure disorder. Anesth Analg 2010;111(3):729–35.

[83] Ahn KS, Kopp SL, Watson JC, et al. Postsurgical inflammatory neuropathy. Reg Anesth Pain Med 2011;36(4):403–5.

[84] Staff NP, Engelstad J, Klein CJ, et al. Post-surgical inflammatory neuropathy. Brain 2010;133(10):2866–80.

[85] Liguori GA. Complications of regional anesthesia: nerve injury and peripheral neural blockade. J Neurosurg Anesthesiol 2004;16(1):84–6.

[86] Seddon HJ. A classification of nerve injuries. Br Med J 1942;2(4260):237–9.

[87] Sunderland S. A classification of peripheral nerve injuries producing loss of function. Brain 1951;74(4):491–516.

[88] Aminoff MJ. Electrophysiologic testing for the diagnosis of peripheral nerve injuries. Anesthesiology 2004;100(5):1298–303.

[89] Horlocker TT, Wedel DJ, Benzon H, et al. Regional anesthesia in the anticoagulated patient: defining the risks (the second ASRA Consensus Conference on Neuraxial Anesthesia and Anticoagulation). Reg Anesth Pain Med 2003;28(3):172–97.

Advances in Anesthesia 29 (2011) 19–37

ADVANCES IN ANESTHESIA

Sugammadex: Past, Present, and Future

James E. Caldwell, MB, ChB

Department of Anesthesia and Perioperative Medicine, University of California, 521 Parnassus Avenue, San Francisco, CA 94143-0648, USA

THE PAST

Ever since the introduction of neuromuscular blocking drugs into anesthesia practice, the mechanism by which the paralytic effect is reversed has been imperfect. Traditional muscle relaxant reversal using inhibitors of anticholinesterase is a flawed process for several reasons. The mechanism of reversal is indirect, the efficacy is limited, rapid reversal of deep block is not possible, and undesirable cardiovascular and autonomic responses occur [1].

Reversal acts indirectly via acetylcholinesterase inhibition

Reversal acts indirectly through inhibition of acetylcholinesterase, the enzyme that metabolizes the endogenous neurotransmitter acetylcholine at the neuromuscular junction. After the administration of an anticholinesterase—whether neostigmine, edrophonium, or pyridostigmine—the metabolism of acetylcholine ceases. As a consequence, the concentration of acetylcholine in the neuromuscular junction increases, and opposes the effect of the muscle relaxant. There is no direct effect on the muscle relaxant itself.

Efficacy of reversal is limited and rapid reversal of deep block is not possible

The efficacy of traditional reversal is limited because when the processes of acetylcholine release, diffusion out of the junction, and reuptake reach equilibrium, the concentration of acetylcholine is at its maximum. The maximum concentration of acetylcholine that can be thus achieved is often insufficient to overcome the effect of the muscle relaxant, and ineffective reversal results [1].

In 1990 Magorian and colleagues [2] neatly demonstrated these limitations of neostigmine. In summary, these investigators showed that neostigmine, 70 µg/kg could not rapidly reverse deep (no response to ulnar nerve stimulation) vecuronium-induced block. More interesting was that a second dose of

---

This work was supported by the University of California Department of Anesthesia and Perioperative Care. The author has nothing to disclose.

E-mail address: caldwell@anesthesia.ucsf.edu

0737-6146/11/$ – see front matter
doi:10.1016/j.aan.2011.07.007

neostigmine, 70 μg/kg, given when recovery from the first dose reached 10% had no further effect on recovery. The second dose of neostigmine neither sped nor slowed subsequent recovery. Therefore before sugammadex, there was no way for clinicians to rapidly reverse what was considered profound levels of neuro-muscular block, namely no train-of-four (TOF) responses of the thumb to electri-cal stimulation of the ulnar nerve [1].

Anticholinesterase reversal has adverse effects

The final set of problems with anticholinesterase drugs is that they have wide-spread undesirable effects at other cholinergic sites. Unopposed muscarinic activity may produce bradycardia, excessive secretions, increased gastrointes-tinal motility, and bronchospasm [1]. Antimuscarinic drugs (glycopyrrolate, atropine) administered to block these effects may produce the opposing effects to excess, for example, tachycardia. Thus the stage was set for a completely new pharmacologic approach to reversal of neuromuscular block, one that would be completely effective against all levels of block and free of autonomic side effects: in short, a drug such as sugammadex [3].

The standard for adequate reversal has been raised

Another force driving the need for a better mechanism for reversal of neuro-muscular block was the redefinition of what constituted an acceptable level of neuromuscular recovery. In the 1970s the concept of the TOF ratio was born and adequate reversal was judged as a TOF ratio of greater than 0.7, because this was associated with adequate vital capacity and inspiratory force [4]. In the late 1990s this dictum was questioned, and current opinion is that subtle but clinically significant effects of muscle relaxants persist unless the TOF ratio is 0.9 or greater and that this should be the new standard [5–8].

As an example, in healthy, nonanesthetized volunteers partially paralyzed with vecuronium and given contrast to swallow, aspiration could occur unless the TOF ratio was at least 0.9 [5,6]. This vulnerability to aspiration was attributable to the disruption of the complex reflex of swallowing (and thus airway protection) induced by even minor degrees of residual block [8]. Another study looked at clinical indices of recovery in healthy volunteers paralyzed with mivacurium [7]. In this study the volunteers felt unsteady when sitting up unless the TOF ratio was 0.9 or more. In addition, diplopia persisted and handgrip strength was reduced even with TOF ratios greater than 0.9. The problem with this new standard for recovery is that it cannot be achieved predictably and reliably with reversal by anticholinesterase administration [9].

Reversal adequacy using anticholinesterase drugs is unpredictable

Because the new standard for adequate reversal is a TOF ratio of 0.9 or greater, the question to ask is: can we reliably achieve this level of recovery with current reversal practices? The answer is no. When reversing cisatracurium-induced block, even when 4 twitches are present and 70 μg/kg neostigmine is given, 26% of patients fail to achieve a TOF ratio of 0.9 or more within 20 minutes [9]. If only one twitch is present when the neostigmine is given, this failure rate rises to 64%. This problem is compounded by the fact that tactile evaluation of the TOF response is very subjective, and the same TOF count can represent a wide range of true neuromuscular block [9]. Fig. 1 shows how any value for tactile TOF count (1–4) can be associated with a wide range of true level of block as measured by a force transducer. For example, at a twitch tension of 12% patients could have a tactile TOF count of 1, 2, 3, or 4 (see Fig. 1).

Discovery of sugammadex

The discovery of sugammadex was serendipitous. Anton Bom, a pharmaceutical chemist with Organon Inc., was performing experiments with rocuronium and needed a drug that would enhance its solubility in the media he was using. He hit on the idea of using cyclodextrins, a group of drugs with a long history in pharmaceutics as solubilizing agents [3,10]. Cyclodextrins are a group of doughnut-shaped sugar molecules consisting of 6 to 8 subunits.

What Bom found was that rocuronium lost its potency when he dissolved it with the cyclodextrin [11]. He could easily have stopped there and moved on to find another solubilizing agent so that he could continue his experiments. Instead he realized that he had a way to "inactivate" rocuronium and thus a radically new mechanism for reversal of neuromuscular block was created. Bom and his group went on to investigate a series of compounds with the purpose of identifying a cyclodextrin that would bind rocuronium with high affinity (ie, irreversibly) [3,10]. Sugammadex (Org 25969) was the compound selected for clinical development. Sugammadex binds

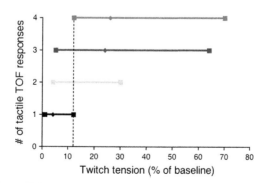

Fig. 1. Twitch tension (X-axis) at which the first, second, third, or fourth tactile response to train-of-four (TOF) stimulation (Y-axis) was detected at the thumb. The poor relationship between tactile count of TOF responses and objective quantitative measurement of neuromuscular block with a force transducer is clear. For example, at a twitch tension or 12% of control, the tactile TOF count felt by the observer in different patients could be 1, 2, 3, or 4. (*Data from* Kirkegaard H, Heier T, Caldwell JE. Efficacy of tactile-guided reversal from cisatracurium-induced neuromuscular block. Anesthesiology 2002;96:45.)

rocuronium 1:1 and essentially decreases the "active" plasma concentration to zero [10,12].

Sugammadex has a lipophilic inner cavity, and the diameter of this cavity is tailored to be an optimal fit for the steroidal nucleus of rocuronium (Fig. 2). In addition, negatively charged hydrophilic carboxyl groups project from the rim of the cyclodextrin molecule [10,12]. These groups, by repelling each other, keep the opening of the cyclodextrin cavity wide, and once the steroidal nucleus is incorporated they close down and lock onto the positively charged quaternary ammonium group of the rocuronium. The rocuronium is thus tightly bound to the cyclodextrin (see Fig. 2).

Sugammadex development pathway

Sugammadex development went along a standard pathway (Fig. 3). In January 2008, the Food and Drug Administration (FDA) took the step of suggesting

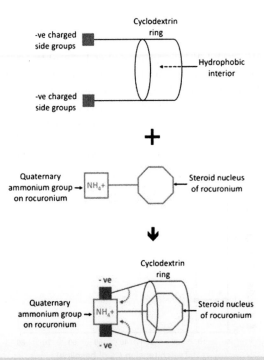

Fig. 2. The interaction of sugammadex and rocuronium. The cyclodextrin has a hydrophobic ring that is conformed optimally to accommodate the steroid nucleus of rocuronium. The ring itself is too small to fit the whole rocuronium molecule, so a method to increase the binding affinity was needed. This increase was accomplished by adding negatively charged side groups, which remain open because of the repulsive force of the negative charges. When a rocuronium molecule enters the cyclodextrin cavity, the negative charge on the side arms is attracted to and locks onto the protruding and positively charged quaternary ammonium group, thus binding the rocuronium with high affinity.

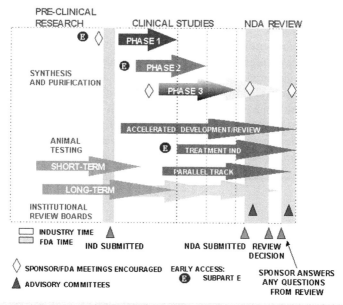

Fig. 3. The development pathway taken by sugammadex when undergoing evaluation by the Food and Drug Administration (FDA). Sugammadex was developed on a parallel track, in that simultaneous studies going on in different countries were used in the submission process to the FDA. At the suggestion of the FDA, sugammadex was placed on a priority (accelerated development) track. At the final expert advisory committee review sugammadex was given a unanimous recommendation for approval. At the final hurdle, the full committee of the FDA, sugammadex was judged "not approvable" because of concerns about possible hypersensitivity reactions. To date sugammadex has been approved in 50 countries worldwide, but not by the FDA. IND, investigational new drug; NDA, new drug application. (This figure is in the public domain at the FDA Center for Drug Evaluation and Research.)

priority (accelerated) review status for sugammadex. A Priority Review designation is given to drugs that offer major advances in treatment, or provide a treatment where no adequate therapy exists. A Priority Review means that the time it takes the FDA to review a new drug application is reduced. The goal for completing a Priority Review is 6 months. Subsequently, a new drug application (NDA) for sugammadex was submitted to the Advisory Committee on Anesthesia and Life Support, and in March 2008 this committee made a unanimous recommendation to the FDA that sugammadex be approved for marketing. The FDA is not bound by this committee's recommendation, but it usually carries significant weight in the final decision of the FDA.

On June 2, 2008, the European Medicines Agency (EMEA) approved sugammadex for clinical release in Europe while in the United States, the FDA decision was awaited with hopeful anticipation. Much to the surprise of those involved in the development of sugammadex, in August 2008 the FDA issued a nonapprovable letter for sugammadex. The reasons given by the FDA for not approving sugammadex centered on concerns about possible hypersensitivity reactions in a small number of study subjects. Subsequently the EMEA re-reviewed the data and saw no reason to change their approval of sugammadex. Since then, sugammadex has been approved in more than 50 countries but remains "not approvable" in the United States, to date the only country that has failed to grant approval when requested. Since the start of development of sugammadex Organon was acquired by Schering-Plough, which was in turn taken over by Merck & Co. The new owner seems committed to continue production and promotion of sugammadex.

THE PRESENT

Before its clinical release we knew that sugammadex, unlike neostigmine, worked well against all degrees of block [13], was unaffected by the use of vapor anesthesia [14], and was free of cardiovascular effects [15]. We knew also that part of its effectiveness was because it inactivated not only the rocuronium in the circulation, but diffused into the neuromuscular junction and inactivated the rocuronium in the area of the acetylcholine receptors themselves [16]. Since its release, sugammadex has been used in a much wider variety of patients than was possible in the clinical trials, and our knowledge of its utility has grown commensurately. As suggested by the clinical trials, it has proved to be effective at reversing all degrees of rocuronium-induced block [17–19].

The difference in efficacy between sugammadex and neostigmine is most noticeable when reversing deep block. Fig. 4 shows a comparison of sugammadex and neostigmine given when only 2 posttetanic twitches are present. Recovery to a TOF ratio of 0.9 or greater was less than 3 minutes in the patient who received sugammadex (4 mg/kg) and greater than 60 minutes in the patient who received neostigmine (70 μg/kg) [20]. Since its widespread release, sugammadex has shown itself effective in a wide variety of clinical situations that were not specifically studied during its development phase.

Sugammadex in specific patient groups

We now know that sugammadex works well both in the elderly [21,22] and in children [23]. It is both efficacious and safe in patients with renal failure [24] or severe cardiac disease [25], and has little effect on the QTc interval [26]. Patients having electroconvulsive therapy require paralysis of rapid onset and short duration, for which succinylcholine has traditionally been the drug of choice. The combination of paralysis with rocuronium and reversal with sugammadex provides both fast onset and rapid recovery, and works well for these patients [27,28]. Rapid reversal of block can be useful in other situations also; for example, sugammadex can rapidly reverse rocuronium during spine surgery to allow for intraoperative neurophysiological monitoring [29].

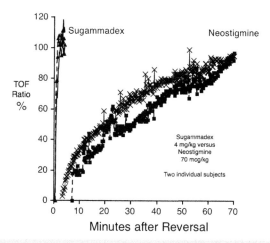

120 ┬
100 ┤ Sugammadex   Neostigmine
TOF
Ratio 80 ┤
%
60 ┤
40 ┤   Sugammadex
                              4 mg/kg versus
                              Neostigmine
                              70 mcg/kg
20 ┤   Two individual subjects
0 ┴
0   10   20   30   40   50   60   70
Minutes after Reversal

Fig. 4. The response in two patients given reversal when there was one posttetanic response. One patient received sugammadex, 4 mg/kg and recovered to a TOF ratio of 0.9 within 3 minutes. The other patient received neostigmine, 70 μg/kg, and took well over an hour to reach a similar level of recovery. This example illustrates that maintaining deep block with rocuronium until the end of the surgical procedure is feasible only if sugammadex is available. (*Data from* Jones RK, Caldwell JE, Brull SJ, et al. Reversal of profound rocuronium-induced blockade with sugammadex: a randomized comparison with neostigmine. Anesthesiology 2008;109:816.)

Sugammadex in patients with neuromuscular disease

Patients with myasthenia gravis are exquisitely sensitive to nondepolarizing blocking drugs, and are at significant risk of inadequate reversal. Sugammadex works very effectively to rapidly restore neuromuscular function in patients with myasthenia gravis paralyzed with rocuronium [30,31]. Response of patients with neuromuscular disease can be difficult to predict, and block difficult to reverse. Because sugammadex results in almost immediate elimination of free and, hence, active rocuronium, the patient is restored to the baseline (prerelaxant) state. This approach has proved useful in the management of patients with myotonic dystrophy [32] and transverse myelitis [33].

Rapid reversal after high-dose rocuronium

Clinicians have always had some degree of trepidation when administering large doses of rocuronium for rapid sequence intubation (RSI), because the patient would remain paralyzed for a considerable length of time and would not recover spontaneous ventilation soon enough to prevent desaturation if their airway could not be managed adequately [34,35]. The availability of sugammadex offers some degree of comfort in the RSI situation. Even high-dose (1.2 mg/kg) rocuronium can be reversed within a few minutes with 16 mg/kg of sugammadex [13]. This treatment does not guarantee recovery of spontaneous ventilation in the "cannot intubate, cannot ventilate" situation, but it will guarantee rapid recovery of neuromuscular function, which can only be to the patient's benefit [36–38]. Such rapid recovery from neuromuscular block was not possible before the introduction of sugammadex, not even with succinylcholine [39].

A special case of RSI is in women having general anesthesia for cesarean section. Succinylcholine has traditionally been the neuromuscular blocking drug used to facilitate rapid tracheal intubation in these patients. Opinion is now shifting toward the use of rocuronium in this situation [40]. A short series of 7 cases showed that while rocuronium, 0.6 mg/kg was sufficient for rapid tracheal intubation, it resulted in significant residual block at the end of the procedure. In all patients the residual paralysis was rapidly reversed with sugammadex, 2 mg/kg [41].

Sugammadex and adverse events

There have been few serious adverse events reported for sugammadex. In one study with 13 volunteers, 96 mg/kg was administered [42], which is 48 times the normal clinical dose and 6 times the maximum clinical dose. One of the volunteers experienced symptoms suggestive of hypersensitivity. A Cochrane meta-analysis found no evidence of a higher rate of adverse events than with placebo [18,43]. To date there has been only one report of a patient who had an apparent allergic reaction to sugammadex, 3.2 mg/kg [44]. An interesting twist on allergic responses is that sugammadex may be useful in the treatment of rocuronium-induced anaphylaxis [45,46].

Given its record of efficacy and safety, one would expect that sugammadex would have replaced neostigmine for routine reversal of rocuronium-induced block. Unfortunately this has not happened, for one overwhelming reason: the price. It appears that the company made a strategic marketing decision to go for a high profit margin on a low volume of sales. This approach has severely limited the use of sugammadex. In Australia, the cost of sugammadex is approximately $1 per milligram. In the United Kingdom, RSI with rocuronium, 1.2 mg/kg followed by sugammadex, 16 mg/kg is 170 times more expensive than using succinylcholine. Because of the high cost, most countries where sugammadex is approved have restricted its use. A quote from the Scottish Medicines Consortium (SMC) illustrates the point: "Sugammadex is not recommended for the routine reversal of neuromuscular blockade induced by rocuronium or vecuronium in adults, children and adolescents as the manufacturer did not present a sufficiently robust economic case to gain acceptance by SMC." A cost-effectiveness analysis suggests that sugammadex can be justified only for use in specialized or emergency situations [47,48].

Because of its high cost, a 200-mg vial costs 78 euros in Germany, 58 pounds in the United Kingdom, and 200 dollars in Australia. Some clinicians have even advocated using very small doses of sugammadex, 0.22 mg/kg, in combination with neostigmine to reverse shallow degrees of residual block [49]. This approach minimizes cost but introduces other potential problems such as using a single-dose vial for multiple patients, and use of several drugs instead of one. There is no doubt that the cost of sugammadex is prohibitive and prevents its more widespread use. Perhaps this situation might change if and when sugammadex becomes a generic drug. The next section outlines the author's personal predictions for what the future might hold if the cost of sugammadex is decreased to a point where it becomes the routine drug for reversal.

THE FUTURE

There are two major questions hanging over the future of sugammadex. One relates to its use in the United States and whether the FDA will eventually approve the drug. The other is what will happen with the pricing of the drug in those countries where it can be used.

The FDA and sugammadex

The reason given by the FDA for not approving sugammadex was concern about possible hypersensitivity reactions. It is unclear what, if anything, will persuade the FDA to change its opinion and approve the drug. The use of sugammadex around the world has not raised any red flags regarding adverse events. In the United States, a study specifically looking at hypersensitivity, the "Sugammadex Hypersensitivity Study (Study P06042)," ClinicalTrials. Gov identifier NCT00988065, has been completed and results are awaited. It is hoped that the FDA will be persuaded to approve sugammadex, and the only concern then will be how the drug is priced.

Sugammadex and cost

If Merck & Co. replicates its current international pricing policy in the United States, sugammadex will cost about $100 for a 200-mg vial [48,49], which is approximately 25 times the cost of reversal with neostigmine and glycopyrrolate [50]. Because the recommended dose for routine reversal when there are 1 or 2 TOF responses is 2 mg/kg, the 200-mg vial will be sufficient for one patient only. Can a cost-benefit case be made for sugammadex at this price?

If the benefit is so great that cost is not an issue then a case can certainly be made. The cost of sugammadex can be justified in cases where no other form of reversal is available. An example would be rapid reversal of rocuronium or vecuronium to restore spontaneous ventilation when airway control cannot be established, the so-called rescue reversal [38,47,51]. Another example might be treating the respiratory failure that occurs when drugs such as magnesium are given in the setting of residual neuromuscular block in the postanesthesia care unit [52]. In a similar vein, sugammadex cost can also be justified if it allows patients to avoid admission to an intensive care unit. For example, a patent whose trachea would remain intubated because of inadequate reversal of block with neostigmine might be given sugammadex and be extubated, and have a less morbid postoperative course [53]. These situations, however, represent only a small fraction of clinical practice. Can sugammadex be justified in more routine practice?

To justify its increased cost, sugammadex would have to decrease expenses in some other area. The single most effective way to decrease cost is to save operating-room time. Whether or not sugammadex can be justified will depend on the cost of the time saved, and how much time can be saved. The cost per minute of operating-room time in the United States is somewhere between $15 and $20 per minute [54]. In theory, if the use of sugammadex reduces operating-room time by 5 minutes it might have paid for itself. For routine reversal from 2 TOF responses, sugammadex produces recovery of TOF ratio = 0.9 in 1.5 minutes versus 18.6 minutes for neostigmine. On the surface this looks like it should justify the cost of sugammadex; however, this is not the whole story.

Most clinicians do not measure the TOF ratio, and extubation is based on clinical criteria. Studies show that the TOF ratio is less than 0.7 when the trachea is extubated at the end of surgery, and in this situation the time advantage of sugammadex over neostigmine is significantly decreased [55]. In addition, tracheal extubation would need to be the rate-limiting step in the time taken to leave the operating room, which usually is not the case. Finally, the full cost of the decreased time would have to be saved, and this is not a realistic expectation [48,56]. If sugammadex is released in the United States with a pricing structure similar to that for other countries, it will be difficult to justify its routine use with simply a cost-benefit analysis.

Justifying sugammadex: quality and safety

There is another argument to justify the use of sugammadex, and that is on the basis of quality and safety. An irreducible incidence of residual neuromuscular block is an inevitable consequence of a reversal strategy based on anticholinesterase drugs [57]. This residual block is not benign, and has measurable adverse effects on the airway and other muscle groups [5–7]. Residual neuromuscular block per se is associated with adverse patient outcomes [5,58,59]. There is even evidence that recovery to a TOF ratio to the new minimum standard of 0.9 leaves patients with measurable impairment of muscle function [60]. The only way to eliminate residual block after administration of rocuronium (or vecuronium) is with sugammadex. It is very difficult to quantify hard cost savings by the elimination of residual block. However, if we assume that it is possible for the use of sugammadex to become routine, then what effect might that have on our practice?

We can maintain profound block until the end of the procedure

Rocuronium will allow profound block to be maintained until the very end of the surgical procedure. Because until now it has been impossible to rapidly reverse deep block, it is a common clinical situation for the surgeon to be requesting a deeper level of muscle relaxation and the anesthesia provider being reluctant to provide this in case reversal proves difficult. There is validity to both sides of the argument. This situation in theory should no longer be a problem because greater doses of rocuronium can be administered and a deeper level of block maintained throughout the procedure. For anesthesia providers, this will require some changes in practice and relearning their techniques of drug administration.

Because of the deeper level of block, parameters for monitoring will also have to change. Because there are no clinically available methods to monitor the diaphragm, clinicians who use nerve stimulators will need to become familiar with using the posttetanic count at the adductor pollicis [61]. However, many anesthesia providers do not use a nerve stimulator and their drug administration has been guided by their experience, clinical acumen, and familiarity with the surgeon's practice [62]. To run deeper levels of block without using a nerve stimulator will require relearning their drug-dosing paradigms.

Sugammadex will allow precise control of rocuronium duration

Sugammadex will allow the duration of action of rocuronium to be precisely tailored to match the clinical needs of any procedure, short or long. An example might be short procedures that require tracheal intubation. Previous possible approaches were to intubate without using a muscle relaxant [63–65], to use succinylcholine, or a small dose, 0.3 to 0.5 mg/kg, of rocuronium [66,67]. Intubating without a relaxant was able to be performed effectively, particularly with propofol and short-acting potent opioids, but it carried the consequence of increased incidences of hypotension and tracheal injury [68]. Succinylcholine's many side effects made clinicians wary of its use, and in pediatrics it should not be used for routine intubation. Finally, intubation assisted with small doses of rocuronium could result in diminished quality of intubation, and still require pharmacologic reversal [66,67]. With sugammadex, a standard intubating dose of rocuronium can be used, and its effects rapidly reversed even if the procedure lasts only a few minutes [13,69].

This exquisite control of the duration of rocuronium has even more implications. Rapid reversal of the effect of rocuronium can be achieved in the scenario of difficulty with airway management and tracheal intubation [13], and may enable rapid return of spontaneous respiration, so-called rescue reversal [51]. It can also make irrelevant the increased variability in the duration of action of rocuronium seen in circumstances such as administration of large doses, organ dysfunction, and treatment of the elderly and the severely obese [70]. Rocuronium will essentially become a drug whose clinical duration and effect can be titrated to exactly match the clinical need. Such facility with control of neuromuscular block has not been available previously.

Benefits of avoiding anticholinesterase reversal

Acetylcholinesterase inhibitors have actions not only at the nicotinic but also at the muscarinic receptors [71]. The unopposed action of neostigmine, for example, would result in severe bradycardia, copious secretions, increased gastrointestinal motility, and bronchospasm [72]. Consequently a drug with antimuscarinic effects, usually atropine or glycopyrrolate, must accompany anticholinesterase drugs.

Even when accompanied by an antimuscarinic drug, neostigmine can result in severe bradycardia in patients with autonomic dysfunction [73], and a case of coronary artery vasospasm provoked by neostigmine has been reported [74]. The antimuscarinic drugs atropine and glycopyrrolate result in impaired parasympathetic control of heart rate with decreased baroreflex sensitivity and high-frequency variability in heart rate [75,76]. It is not always possible to balance exactly the muscarinic effects of the anticholinesterase and the dose of atropine or glycopyrrolate. As a result, changes in heart rate commonly occur with reversal [77–79]. Clinicians who might omit pharmacologic reversal because of these potential adverse effects may now be comfortable reversing the rocuronium effect with sugammadex.

Other concerns with the use of neostigmine, such as possible increase in the rate of postoperative nausea and vomiting [80] or breakdown of colonic anastomoses [81], will no longer be issues with sugammadex.

Will we still need muscle relaxants other than rocuronium?

With sugammadex the duration of rocuronium action can be tailored to any clinical situation and its rapid and complete reversal guaranteed. Does this suggest that a case be made for eliminating the use of other relaxants? It is certainly cost-advantageous for a pharmacy to decrease the number of drugs on its formulary. So what drugs might we eliminate?

The first to consider for elimination is vecuronium. Because sugammadex is less efficacious with vecuronium than rocuronium, and vecuronium has an active metabolite, there seems very little reason to keep vecuronium [82,83]. Second, the benefits of the rocuronium/sugammadex combination do not exist with the benzylisoquinolinium relaxants atracurium, cisatracurium, and mivacurium. Should the availability of sugammadex lead to the decreased use of these drugs? This question is difficult to answer, and will depend on factors such as why the clinician uses the other drug in the first place. Is it because of perceived problems with rocuronium such as variability of duration, or concern over possible severe allergic reactions? Sugammadex can remove the former objection to rocuronium, but not the latter.

Before sugammadex, cisatracurium had an advantage over rocuronium in that it had a less variable duration of action [70,84], and its recovery was less affected by impaired organ function. The availability of sugammadex will eliminate these advantages. In a direct comparison, reversal with sugammadex-rocuronium was almost 5 times faster than with the cisatracurium-neostigmine combination, 1.9 versus 9.0 minutes [85]. There is one situation in which it may be necessary to retain the availability of cisatracurium. If, after reversal of rocuronium with sugammadex, a patient needs to be urgently reintubated, then cisatracurium can be used because is not affected by sugammadex.

Mivacurium is still in common use in some countries, mostly because of its short duration of action [86,87]. However, even with its short duration of action mivacurium can have a high incidence (about 10%) of residual block unless its action is pharmacologically reversed [88]. In comparison, rocuronium already has faster onset than mivacurium, and with the use of sugammadex it can be made to have a short duration of action, thus to be free of residual block and the adverse effects of anticholinesterase reversal. Potentially, therefore, with the exception of cisatracurium for urgent reintubation, benzylisoquinolinium drugs could be eliminated from clinical use.

Will we still need succinylcholine?

To answer this question requires that we define why succinylcholine is necessary in the first place. To begin, succinylcholine is unique in having a fast onset and short duration of action. Second, no other relaxant provides better conditions for tracheal intubation, although rocuronium in large doses (1.2 mg/kg) is almost as good [89,90]. Finally, succinylcholine dosing is flexible and there is little penalty in terms of prolonged duration for using increased doses. Because of these attributes, succinylcholine has been used for RSI, intubation for short procedures, intubation for longer procedures whereby no further relaxation is required, and intubation in patients for whom dose calculations for rocuronium are difficult, for example, the morbidly obese [91].

The advent of sugammadex has rendered succinylcholine redundant for essentially all of these situations. For RSI, a large dose of rocuronium can be used with similar quality of intubation as succinylcholine [90], and without risk of prolonged duration [13,69]. Procedures, either short or long, requiring paralysis just for tracheal intubation are amenable to use of rocuronium [69,92]. It is difficult to see where succinylcholine will be needed except in one circumstance, the same as already described for cisatracurium, that is, reintubation after reversal with sugammadex. In conclusion, succinylcholine will continue to have a place, but one that is much diminished where rocuronium and sugammadex are used.

Implications of sugammadex for neuromuscular function monitoring

There are two principal indications for neuromuscular monitoring: one is to guide intraoperative dosing of relaxant, the second is to assess adequacy of reversal. For the first, where monitoring is used, the tactile TOF count at the adductor pollicis has been standard practice for many years. However, if sugammadex promotes the use of deeper levels of block, the TOF response is an inadequate monitoring modality for monitoring of this deeper block [61].

Compared with the adductor pollicis, the diaphragm and larynx require a plasma concentration 1.6 to 1.8 times higher to achieve the same level of block [93–95]. This concentration of relaxant will completely abolish the TOF responses at the thumb, so the posttetanic count (PTC) will need to be used [61]. This stimulation modality is available on all modern nerve stimulators for operating-room use, and allows the clinician to monitor the depth of block required for paralysis of the diaphragm and larynx. The PTC can also guide sugammadex administration at the end of the procedure. If only 1 or 2 posttetanic responses are present, the appropriate dose of sugammadex is 4 mg/kg [20,96].

Despite the many recommendations by experts that encourage the use clinical neuromuscular monitoring, evidence that it is of benefit in decreasing residual paralysis is lacking [97]. Monitoring can only reliably document adequate recovery if it measures and displays the TOF ratio. Clinical assessment of TOF ratio, tetanic fade, or even double-burst fade does not have the sensitivity to reliably detect TOF of below 0.7, much less below 0.9 [98].

Quantitative measurement of TOF ratio using acceleromyography (AMG) is clinically available [98], and can detect even minor degrees of residual block. Unfortunately, detecting the block does not mean that it can be reversed. If the patient already has had a full dose of anticholinesterase then no more can be done to accelerate recovery [2]. How will sugammadex alter neuromuscular monitoring? The answer is that the cost of the drug will possibly drive monitoring at the end of the case to determine the minimum dose that can be given to achieve an acceptable degree of recovery, for example, TOF ratio = 1.0 [48,50,56,99,100].

Sugammadex dosing recommendations

The recommendations for dosing sugammadex are 2 mg/kg at 2 TOF responses, 4 mg/kg for a level of 2 posttetanic responses, and 16 mg/kg for immediate reversal of a large dose of rocuronium (Table 1). If the drug is very expensive, clinicians may start to titrate their dosing against the TOF recovery on the AMG and stop administration when the TOF ratio is 1.0. In doing this they need to keep in mind that if underdosed, sugammadex will not be effective [101]. Alternatively, if cost is not an issue, clinicians will simply administer a large dose, confident in the drugs affect, and not monitor reversal at all. Sugammadex could conceivably eliminate the need for monitoring of reversal in patients receiving rocuronium [102].

Table 1
Dose recommendations and estimated cost of sugammadex in different clinical reversal scenarios

Scenario	Sugammadex dose (mg/kg)	Number of vials (200 mg) (for 80 kg patient)	Estimated cost in US$ (50 cents/mg)
PTC = 1 or 2	16	7	700
PTC = 1 or 2	4	2	200
TOF count = 1 or 2	2	1	100
TOF count = 4	1	1 (0.5)	50[a]
TOF ratio ≥0.5	0.22	1 (0.2)	20[a]

Abbreviations: PTC, posttetanic count; TOF, train-of-four.
[a]Cost estimate is for contents of one 200-mg vial of sugammadex divided up between several patients.

References

[1] Caldwell JE. Clinical limitations of acetylcholinesterase antagonists. J Crit Care 2009; 24:21.

[2] Magorian TT, Lynam DP, Caldwell J, et al. Can early administration of neostigmine, in single or divided doses, alter the course of neuromuscular recovery from a vecuronium-induced neuromuscular blockade? Anesthesiology 1990;73:410.

[3] Bom A, Bradley M, Cameron K, et al. A novel concept of reversing neuromuscular block: chemical encapsulation of rocuronium bromide by a cyclodextrin-based synthetic host. Angew Chem Int Ed Engl 2002;41:266.

[4] Brand JB, Cullen DJ, Wilson NE, et al. Spontaneous recovery from nondepolarizing neuromuscular blockade: correlation between clinical and evoked responses. Anesth Analg 1977;56:55.

[5] Eriksson LI. Residual neuromuscular blockade. Incidence and relevance. Anaesthesist 2000;49(Suppl 1):S18.

[6] Eriksson LI, Sundman E, Olsson R, et al. Functional assessment of the pharynx at rest and during swallowing in partially paralyzed humans: simultaneous videomanometry and mechanomyography of awake human volunteers. Anesthesiology 1997;87:1035.

[7] Kopman AF, Yee PS, Neuman GG. Relationship of the train-of-four fade ratio to clinical signs and symptoms of residual paralysis in awake volunteers. Anesthesiology 1997;86:765.

[8] Sundman E, Witt H, Olsson R, et al. The incidence and mechanisms of pharyngeal and upper esophageal dysfunction in partially paralyzed humans: pharyngeal videoradiography and simultaneous manometry after atracurium. Anesthesiology 2000;92:977.

[9] Kirkegaard H, Heier T, Caldwell JF Ffficacy of tactile-guided reversal from cisatracurium-induced neuromuscular block. Anesthesiology 2002;96:45.

[10] Adam JM, Bennett DJ, Bom A, et al. Cyclodextrin-derived host molecules as reversal agents for the neuromuscular blocker rocuronium bromide: synthesis and structure-activity relationships. J Med Chem 2002;45:1086.

[11] Booij LH. Cyclodextrins and the emergence of sugammadex. Anaesthesia 2009; 64(Suppl 1):31.

[12] Tarver GJ, Grove SJ, Buchanan K, et al. 2-O-substituted cyclodextrins as reversal agents for the neuromuscular blocker rocuronium bromide. Bioorg Med Chem 2002;10:1819.

[13] Puhringer FK, Rex C, Sielenkamper AW, et al. Reversal of profound, high-dose rocuronium-induced neuromuscular blockade by sugammadex at two different time points: an international, multicenter, randomized, dose-finding, safety assessor-blinded, phase II trial. Anesthesiology 2008;109:188.

[14] Vanacker BF, Vermeyen KM, Struys MM, et al. Reversal of rocuronium-induced neuromuscular block with the novel drug sugammadex is equally effective under maintenance anesthesia with propofol or sevoflurane. Anesth Analg 2007;104:563.

[15] Cammu G, De Kam PJ, Demeyer I, et al. Safety and tolerability of single intravenous doses of sugammadex administered simultaneously with rocuronium or vecuronium in healthy volunteers. Br J Anaesth 2008;100:373.

[16] Nigrovic V, Bhatt SB, Amann A. Simulation of the reversal of neuromuscular block by sequestration of the free molecules of the muscle relaxant. J Pharmacokinet Pharmacodyn 2007;34:771.

[17] Duvaldestin P, Plaud B. Sugammadex in anesthesia practice. Expert Opin Pharmacother 2010;11:2759.

[18] Abrishami A, Ho J, Wong J, et al. Cochrane corner: sugammadex, a selective reversal medication for preventing postoperative residual neuromuscular blockade. Anesth Analg 2010;110:1239.

[19] Yang LP, Keam SJ. Sugammadex: a review of its use in anaesthetic practice. Drugs 2009;69:919.

[20] Jones RK, Caldwell JE, Brull SJ, et al. Reversal of profound rocuronium-induced blockade with sugammadex: a randomized comparison with neostigmine. Anesthesiology 2008;109:816.

[21] McDonagh DL, Benedict PE, Kovac AL, et al. Efficacy, safety, and pharmacokinetics of sugammadex for the reversal of rocuronium-induced neuromuscular blockade in elderly patients. Anesthesiology 2011;114:318.

[22] Suzuki T, Kitajima O, Ueda K, et al. Reversibility of rocuronium-induced profound neuromuscular block with sugammadex in younger and older patients. Br J Anaesth 2011;106(6):823–6.

[23] Plaud B, Meretoja O, Hofmockel R, et al. Reversal of rocuronium-induced neuromuscular blockade with sugammadex in pediatric and adult surgical patients. Anesthesiology 2009;110:284.

[24] Staals LM, Snoeck MM, Driessen JJ, et al. Reduced clearance of rocuronium and sugammadex in patients with severe to end-stage renal failure: a pharmacokinetic study. Br J Anaesth 2010;104:31.

[25] Dahl V, Pendeville PE, Hollmann MW, et al. Safety and efficacy of sugammadex for the reversal of rocuronium-induced neuromuscular blockade in cardiac patients undergoing noncardiac surgery. Eur J Anaesthesiol 2009;26:874.

[26] de Kam PJ, van Kuijk J, Prohn M, et al. Effects of sugammadex doses up to 32 mg/kg alone or in combination with rocuronium or vecuronium on QTc prolongation: a thorough QTc study. Clin Drug Investig 2010;30:599.

[27] Batistaki C, Kesidis K, Apostolaki S, et al. Rocuronium antagonized by sugammadex for series of electroconvulsive therapy (ECT) in a patient with pseudocholinesterase deficiency. J ECT 2011.

[28] Hoshi H, Kadoi Y, Kamiyama J, et al. Use of rocuronium-sugammadex, an alternative to succinylcholine, as a muscle relaxant during electroconvulsive therapy. J Anesth 2011;25(2):286–90.

[29] Reid S, Shields MO, Luney SR. Use of sugammadex for reversal of neuromuscular blockade in 2 patients requiring intraoperative neurophysiological monitoring. J Neurosurg Anesthesiol 2011;23:56.

[30] Unterbuchner C, Fink H, Blobner M. The use of sugammadex in a patient with myasthenia gravis. Anaesthesia 2010.

[31] Petrun AM, Mekis D, Kamenik M. Successful use of rocuronium and sugammadex in a patient with myasthenia. Eur J Anaesthesiol 2010;27:917.

[32] Matsuki Y, Hirose M, Tabata M, et al. The use of sugammadex in a patient with myotonic dystrophy. Eur J Anaesthesiol 2011;28:145.

[33] Weekes G, Hayes N, Bowen M. Reversal of prolonged rocuronium neuromuscular blockade with sugammadex in an obstetric patient with transverse myelitis. Int J Obstet Anesth 2010;19:333.

[34] Naguib M, Samarkandi AH, Abdullah K, et al. Succinylcholine dosage and apnea-induced hemoglobin desaturation in patients. Anesthesiology 2005;102:35.

[35] Heier T, Feiner JR, Lin J, et al. Hemoglobin desaturation after succinylcholine-induced apnea: a study of the recovery of spontaneous ventilation in healthy volunteers. Anesthesiology 2001;94:754.

[36] Dada A, Dunsire F. Can sugammadex save a patient in a simulated 'cannot intubate, cannot ventilate' scenario? Anaesthesia 2011;66:141.

[37] Rex C, Bergner UA, Puhringer FK. Sugammadex: a selective relaxant-binding agent providing rapid reversal. Curr Opin Anaesthesiol 2010;23:461.

[38] McTernan CN, Rapeport DA, Ledowski T. Successful use of rocuronium and sugammadex in an anticipated difficult airway scenario. Anaesth Intensive Care 2010;38:390.

[39] Lee C, Jahr JS, Candiotti KA, et al. Reversal of profound neuromuscular block by sugammadex administered three minutes after rocuronium: a comparison with spontaneous recovery from succinylcholine. Anesthesiology 2009;110:1020.

[40] Sharp LM, Levy DM. Rapid sequence induction in obstetrics revisited. Curr Opin Anaesthesiol 2009;22:357.

[41] Puhringer FK, Kristen P, Rex C. Sugammadex reversal of rocuronium-induced neuromuscular block in Caesarean section patients: a series of seven cases. Br J Anaesth 2010;105:657.

[42] Peeters PA, van den Heuvel MW, van Heumen E, et al. Safety, tolerability and pharmacokinetics of sugammadex using single high doses (up to 96 mg/kg) in healthy adult subjects: a randomized, double-blind, crossover, placebo-controlled, single-centre study. Clin Drug Investig 2010;30:867.

[43] Abrishami A, Ho J, Wong J, et al. Sugammadex, a selective reversal medication for preventing postoperative residual neuromuscular blockade. Cochrane Database Syst Rev 2009;CD007362.

[44] Menendez-Ozcoidi L, Ortiz-Gomez JR, Olaguibel-Ribero JM, et al. Allergy to low dose sugammadex. Anaesthesia 2011;66:217.

[45] McDonnell NJ, Pavy TJ, Green LK, et al. Sugammadex in the management of rocuronium-induced anaphylaxis. Br J Anaesth 2011;106:199.

[46] Jones PM, Turkstra TP. Mitigation of rocuronium-induced anaphylaxis by sugammadex: the great unknown. Anaesthesia 2010;65:89.

[47] Chambers D, Paulden M, Paton F, et al. Sugammadex for reversal of neuromuscular block after rapid sequence intubation: a systematic review and economic assessment. Br J Anaesth 2010;105:568.

[48] Paton F, Paulden M, Chambers D, et al. Sugammadex compared with neostigmine/glycopyrrolate for routine reversal of neuromuscular block: a systematic review and economic evaluation. Br J Anaesth 2010;105:558.

[49] Schaller SJ, Fink H, Ulm K, et al. Sugammadex and neostigmine dose-finding study for reversal of shallow residual neuromuscular block. Anesthesiology 2010;113:1054.

[50] Kopman AF. Neostigmine versus sugammadex: which, when, and how much? Anesthesiology 2010;113:1010.

[51] Mirakhur RK, Shields MO, de Boer HD. Sugammadex and rescue reversal. Anaesthesia 2011;66:140.

[52] Fawcett WJ, Stone JP. Recurarization in the recovery room following the use of magnesium sulphate. Br J Anaesth 2003;91:435.

[53] Porter MV, Paleologos MS. The use of rocuronium in a patient with cystic fibrosis and end-stage lung disease made safe by sugammadex reversal. Anaesth Intensive Care 2011;39:299.

[54] Macario A. What does one minute of operating room time cost? J Clin Anesth 2010;22:233.

[55] Sacan O, White PF, Tufanogullari B, et al. Sugammadex reversal of rocuronium-induced neuromuscular blockade: a comparison with neostigmine-glycopyrrolate and edrophonium-atropine. Anesth Analg 2007;104:569.

[56] Chambers D, Paulden M, Paton F, et al. Sugammadex for the reversal of muscle relaxation in general anaesthesia: a systematic review and economic assessment. Health Technol Assess 2010;14:1.

[57] Debaene B, Plaud B, Dilly MP, et al. Residual paralysis in the PACU after a single intubating dose of nondepolarizing muscle relaxant with an intermediate duration of action. Anesthesiology 2003;98:1042.

[58] Murphy GS, Brull SJ. Residual neuromuscular block: lessons unlearned. Part I: definitions, incidence, and adverse physiologic effects of residual neuromuscular block. Anesth Analg 2010;111:120.

[59] Murphy GS, Szokol JW, Marymont JH, et al. Residual neuromuscular blockade and critical respiratory events in the postanesthesia care unit. Anesth Analg 2008;107:130.

[60] Eikermann M, Gerwig M, Hasselmann C, et al. Impaired neuromuscular transmission after recovery of the train-of-four ratio. Acta Anaesthesiol Scand 2007;51:226.

[61] Bonsu AK, Viby-Mogensen J, Fernando PU, et al. Relationship of post-tetanic count and train-of-four response during intense neuromuscular blockade caused by atracurium. Br J Anaesth 1987;59:1089.

[62] Fuchs-Buder T, Fink H, Hofmockel R, et al. Application of neuromuscular monitoring in Germany. Anaesthesist 2008;57:908 [in German].

[63] Alexander R, Booth J, Olufolabi AJ, et al. Comparison of remifentanil with alfentanil or suxamethonium following propofol anaesthesia for tracheal intubation. Anaesthesia 1999;54:1032.

[64] Joo HS, Perks WJ, Belo SE. Sevoflurane with remifentanil allows rapid tracheal intubation without neuromuscular blocking agents. Can J Anaesth 2001;48:646.

[65] Scheller MS, Zornow MH, Saidman LJ. Tracheal intubation without the use of muscle relaxants: A technique using propofol and varying doses of alfentanil. Anesth Analg 1992;75:788.

[66] Kopman AF, Klewicka MM, Neuman GG. Reexamined: the recommended endotracheal intubating dose for nondepolarizing neuromuscular blockers of rapid onset. Anesth Analg 2001;93:954.

[67] Barclay K, Eggers K, Asai T. Low-dose rocuronium improves conditions for tracheal intubation after induction of anaesthesia with propofol and alfentanil. Br J Anaesth 1997;78:92.

[68] Mencke T, Echternach M, Kleinschmidt S, et al. Laryngeal morbidity and quality of tracheal intubation: a randomized controlled trial. Anesthesiology 2003;98:1049.

[69] Sparr HJ, Vermeyen KM, Beaufort AM, et al. Early reversal of profound rocuronium-induced neuromuscular blockade by sugammadex in a randomized multicenter study: efficacy, safety, and pharmacokinetics. Anesthesiology 2007;106:935.

[70] Maybauer DM, Geldner G, Blobner M, et al. Incidence and duration of residual paralysis at the end of surgery after multiple administrations of cisatracurium and rocuronium. Anaesthesia 2007;62:12.

[71] Barth CD, Ebert TJ. Autonomic nervous system. In: Hemmings HC, Hopkins PM, editors. Foundations of anesthesia. Philadelphia: Elsevier; 2006. p. 403.

[72] Clutton RE, Boyd C, Flora R, et al. Autonomic and cardiovascular effects of neuromuscular blockade antagonism in the dog. Vet Surg 1992;21:68.

[73] Triantafillou AN, Tsueda K, Berg J, et al. Refractory bradycardia after reversal of muscle relaxant in a diabetic with vagal neuropathy. Anesth Analg 1986;65:1237.

[74] Kido K, Mizuta K, Mizuta F, et al. Coronary vasospasm during the reversal of neuromuscular block using neostigmine. Acta Anaesthesiol Scand 2005;49:1395.

[75] Muir AW, Houston J, Marshall RJ, et al. A comparison of the neuromuscular blocking and autonomic effects of two new short-acting muscle relaxants with those of succinylcholine in the anesthetized cat and pig. Anesthesiology 1989;70:533.

[76] van Vlymen JM, Parlow JL. The effects of reversal of neuromuscular blockade on autonomic control in the perioperative period. Anesth Analg 1997;84:148.

[77] Cozanitis DA, Dundee JW, Merrett JD, et al. Evaluation of glycopyrrolate and atropine as adjuncts to reversal of non-depolarizing neuromuscular blocking agents in a "true-to-life" situation. Br J Anaesth 1980;52:85.

[78] Mirakhur RK, Dundee JW, Clarke RS. Glycopyrrolate-neostigmine mixture for antagonism of neuromuscular block: comparison with atropine-neostigmine mixture. Br J Anaesth 1977;49:825.

[79] Mirakhur RK, Dundee JW, Jones CJ, et al. Reversal of neuromuscular blockade: dose determination studies with atropine and glycopyrrolate given before or in a mixture with neostigmine. Anesth Analg 1981;60:557.

[80] Lovstad RZ, Thagaard KS, Berner NS, et al. Neostigmine 50 microg kg(-1) with glycopyrrolate increases postoperative nausea in women after laparoscopic gynaecological surgery. Acta Anaesthesiol Scand 2001;45:495.

[81] Olivieri L, Pierdominici S, Testa G, et al. Dehiscence of intestinal anastomoses and anaesthesia. Ital J Surg Sci 1988;18:217.

[82] Puhringer FK, Gordon M, Demeyer I, et al. Sugammadex rapidly reverses moderate rocuronium- or vecuronium-induced neuromuscular block during sevoflurane anaesthesia: a dose-response relationship. Br J Anaesth 2010;105:610.

[83] Staals LM, van Egmond J, Driessen JJ, et al. Sugammadex reverses neuromuscular block induced by 3-desacetyl-vecuronium, an active metabolite of vecuronium, in the anaesthetised rhesus monkey. Eur J Anaesthesiol 2011;28(4):265–72.

[84] Adamus M, Belohlavek R, Koutna J, et al. Cisatracurium vs. rocuronium: a prospective, comparative, randomized study in adult patients under total intravenous anaesthesia. Biomed Pap Med Fac Univ Palacky Olomouc Czech Repub 2006;150:333.

[85] Flockton EA, Mastronardi P, Hunter JM, et al. Reversal of rocuronium-induced neuromuscular block with sugammadex is faster than reversal of cisatracurium-induced block with neostigmine. Br J Anaesth 2008;100:622.

[86] Fink H, Geldner G, Fuchs-Buder T, et al. Muscle relaxants in Germany 2005: a comparison of application customs in hospitals and private practices. Anaesthesist 2006;55:668 [in German].

[87] Nauheimer D, Fink H, Fuchs-Buder T, et al. Muscle relaxant use for tracheal intubation in pediatric anaesthesia: a survey of clinical practice in Germany. Paediatr Anaesth 2009;19:225.

[88] Bevan DR, Kahwaji R, Ansermino JM, et al. Residual block after mivacurium with or without edrophonium reversal in adults and children. Anesthesiology 1996;84:362.

[89] Karcioglu O, Arnold J, Topacoglu H, et al. Succinylcholine or rocuronium? A meta-analysis of the effects on intubation conditions. Int J Clin Pract 2006;60:1638.

[90] Perry JJ, Lee JS, Sillberg VA, et al. Rocuronium versus succinylcholine for rapid sequence induction intubation. Cochrane Database Syst Rev 2008;CD002788.

[91] Meyhoff CS, Lund J, Jenstrup MT, et al. Should dosing of rocuronium in obese patients be based on ideal or corrected body weight? Anesth Analg 2009;109:787.

[92] Suy K, Morias K, Cammu G, et al. Effective reversal of moderate rocuronium- or vecuronium-induced neuromuscular block with sugammadex, a selective relaxant binding agent. Anesthesiology 2007;106:283.

[93] Bragg P, Fisher DM, Shi J, et al. Comparison of twitch depression of the adductor pollicis and the respiratory muscles. Pharmacodynamic modeling without plasma concentrations. Anesthesiology 1994;80:310.

[94] Cantineau JP, Porte F, d'Honneur G, et al. Neuromuscular effects of rocuronium on the diaphragm and adductor pollicis muscles in anesthetized patients. Anesthesiology 1994;81:585.

[95] Donati F, Meistelman C, Plaud B. Vecuronium neuromuscular blockade at the diaphragm, the orbicularis oculi, and adductor pollicis muscles. Anesthesiology 1990;73:870.

[96] Groudine SB, Soto R, Lien C, et al. A randomized, dose-finding, phase II study of the selective relaxant binding drug, Sugammadex, capable of safely reversing profound rocuronium-induced neuromuscular block. Anesth Analg 2007;104:555.

[97] Naguib M, Kopman AF, Ensor JE. Neuromuscular monitoring and postoperative residual curarisation: a meta-analysis. Br J Anaesth 2007;98:302.

[98] Capron F, Fortier LP, Racine S, et al. Tactile fade detection with hand or wrist stimulation using train-of-four, double-burst stimulation, 50-hertz tetanus, 100-hertz tetanus, and acceleromyography. Anesth Analg 2006;102:1578.

[99] Kopman AF. Sugammadex dose requirements at posttetanic counts of 1 to 2: cost implications. Anesth Analg 2010;110:1753.

[100] Debaene B, Meistelman C. Indications and clinical use of sugammadex. Ann Fr Anesth Reanim 2009;28(Suppl 2):S57 [in French].

[101] Fuchs-Buder T. Less is not always more: sugammadex and the risk of under-dosing. Eur J Anaesthesiol 2010;27:849.

[102] Fuchs-Buder T, Meistelman C. Monitoring of neuromuscular block and prevention of residual paralysis. Ann Fr Anesth Reanim 2009;28(Suppl 2):S46 [in French].

Advances in Anesthesia 29 (2011) 39–58

ADVANCES IN ANESTHESIA

ELSEVIER
MOSBY

Occupational Hazards for the Pregnant Anesthesia Provider

Cari L. Meyer, MD

Department of Anesthesiology, University of Wisconsin School of Medicine and Public Health, 600 Highland Avenue, B6/318 CSC, Madison, WI 53792, USA

I n today's operating rooms, almost 30% of anesthesiologists, 36% of anesthesiology residents, and 51% of certified registered nurse anesthetists (CRNAs) are women [1,2]. Many of these women are of childbearing age, and experience at least 1 pregnancy during their career. It is important for them, their colleagues, and their employers to be aware of the possible occupational hazards that exist for pregnant anesthesia providers. This review covers the occupational hazards of waste anesthetic gases, radiation, magnetic resonance imaging (MRI), medications and chemicals in the operating room, and infectious patients. Theoretic risks, animal evidence, and human evidence for risk are presented, and measures to minimize risk are discussed.

First, we must have an understanding of the outcomes and the baseline risks that exist. The adverse pregnancy outcomes that are considered are spontaneous abortions, premature births, and birth defects. Spontaneous abortion, or miscarriage, is defined as the loss of a nonviable fetus, and most of these events occur in the first trimester. In the general population, 10% to 20% of women who know they are pregnant miscarry before 20 weeks of gestation [3]. For women more than 40 years old, the miscarriage rate increases to 35% to 50%, and for those using assisted reproductive technologies the number is even higher. A premature birth is one that occurs before 37 weeks of gestation, and the overall premature birth rate is 12.3% in the United States [4]. As for birth defects, these are congenital anomalies that can be chromosomal or nonchromosomal in origin. In the general population, there is a 3% to 4% background rate for birth defects, and the incidence increases with advanced maternal age and the use of assisted reproductive technologies [5].

Clearly there is risk associated with all pregnancies, and all adverse pregnancy outcomes in anesthesia providers cannot be attributed to occupational exposures. The goal of this review is to present information that helps women protect themselves in the workplace so they are not at any increased risk because of their profession.

E-mail address: cmeyer@wisc.edu

0737-6146/11/$ – see front matter
doi:10.1016/j.aan.2011.07.006

ANESTHETIC GASES IN PREGNANCY

Concern about occupational exposure to inhalational anesthetics has existed for many years. This concern is based on basic science, animal research, and human epidemiologic studies. In 1981, the American Society of Anesthesiologists (ASA) published its first booklet, *Waste Anesthetics in Operating Room Air: A Suggested Program to Reduce Personnel Exposure*, written by the ASA Committee on the Effects of Trace Anesthetic Agents on Health of Operating Room Personnel [6]. In 1999, this booklet was revised and updated when the Task Force on Trace Anesthetic Gases of the ASA Committee on Occupational Health released the booklet titled *Waste Anesthetic Gases: Information for Management in Anesthetizing Areas and the Postanesthesia Care Unit* [7]. Most recently, in 2005 the ASA Task Force released an educational video *Facts About Waste Anesthetic Gases*. The materials published by the ASA contain an analysis of the subject and present critical descriptions of the important papers. They make several recommendations to minimize trace concentrations of waste anesthetic gases in all anesthetizing areas, advocate for scavenging of waste anesthetic gases, and outline appropriate work practices. The overall conclusion of the Task Force, based on currently available studies, is that there is no association between occupational exposure to trace levels of waste anesthetic gases in properly scavenged operating rooms and adverse health effects in pregnant women.

Nitrous oxide

Nitrous oxide has a mechanism of action that could be expected to lead to teratogenesis. Nitrous oxide interacts with vitamin B_{12}, the coenzyme for methionine synthase (also known as 5-methyltetrahydrofolate homocysteine methyltransferase). This interaction leads to a decrease in the activity of methionine synthase, and a decrease in methionine production. The activated form of methionine, S-adenosylmethionine, is the principal substrate for methylation in many biochemical reactions, including assembly of the myelin sheath, methyl substitutions in neurotransmitters, and DNA synthesis in rapidly proliferating tissues. So nitrous oxide, by way of inhibition of methionine synthase, causes an inhibition of the synthesis of thymidine and DNA [8]. Because fetal development is a time of rapid DNA synthesis, this has been shown to be a particularly vulnerable time. Studies from the 1970s and 1980s reported that when pregnant rats were exposed to nitrous oxide, significant decreases in DNA synthesis and content were observed in the embryos [9,10]. Interference with DNA synthesis has also been report in humans who have had prolonged exposures to nitrous oxide [11,12].

How are these effects manifested clinically? Several animal studies have reported reproductive and developmental abnormalities in pregnant rats exposed to nitrous oxide. A few studies showed growth retardation and malformations, such as ocular, limb, rib, and vertebral defects in the offspring of rats who had prolonged exposures to nitrous oxide during pregnancy [13,14]. Studies have shown an increase in fetal resorptions, or spontaneous abortions, in exposed rats [15–20]. Although the levels of nitrous oxide and the times of exposure were high in many of the early studies, later studies strove to approximate the exposure that health care workers might experience in unscavenged operating rooms. Even with the lower levels and shorter durations, chronic repeated exposure to nitrous oxide resulted in increases in spontaneous abortions in rats.

The human studies regarding nitrous oxide exposure are primarily retrospective and epidemiologic in nature. Several investigators have reported that women with occupational exposure before and during their pregnancies had 1.5 to 2 times the risk of spontaneous abortion than nonexposed cohorts. These studies were performed in the 1970s and 1980s, and most of these were conducted as mail surveys of anesthesiologists [21–23], operating room nurses [21,24], and dentists and dental assistants [25]. The results of these studies have been contradicted by smaller studies that have not found an increase in the rates of spontaneous abortion [26,27]. The methodology and validity of the studies have also been questioned [28,29]. The studies all have similar designs, and may therefore all suffer from the same design flaws. Potential problems include the lack of criteria for exposure or outcome, poor survey response rates, selection and recall bias, a lack of validation of the outcomes, and a lack of control for potentially confounding variables.

Another important point is that the study participants in the 1970s and 1980s were often working in environments that did not have modern scavenging of waste anesthetic gases. In the 1990s, Rowland and colleagues [30] addressed this difference by conducting studies of dental assistants working with nitrous oxide in scavenged versus unscavenged settings. These investigators found that female dental assistants exposed to unscavenged nitrous oxide had a significantly increased risk of reduced fertility compared with nonexposed female dental assistants. When dental assistants used scavenging systems during nitrous oxide administration, the probability of conception was not significantly different from that of nonexposed assistants. The study also revealed that the mean time to conception was significantly longer for women who worked with unscavenged nitrous oxide than it was for women who worked with scavenged nitrous oxide or for nonexposed women. The same group later showed that women who worked with nitrous oxide in the absence of scavenging equipment had an increased risk of spontaneous abortion [31]. This finding was not observed among workers in offices where scavenging equipment was in use.

Although there are some issues with study design and selection bias in the older studies, the evidence regarding potential health risks from exposure to nitrous oxide in unscavenged environments suggests that clinicians should be concerned. In addition, there are biologic mechanisms that add to the concern that high levels of nitrous oxide may have reproductive risks. However, proper scavenging can significantly decrease exposure levels, and seems to mitigate the risk. The ASA believes that scavenging is important, and after a thorough review, has stated that there is no association between occupational exposure to trace levels of nitrous oxide in properly scavenged operating rooms and adverse health effects in pregnant women.

Halogenated agents

The history of the halogenated agents is similar to that of nitrous oxide. Since 1970, there have been reports that halothane and isoflurane can have embry-olethal and teratogenic effects in rats, mice, and hamsters [32–34]. The early studies used high exposure levels for prolonged periods, conditions that are dissimilar to human occupational exposures. Later studies, carried out in the mid-1980s, used levels of isoflurane that are more comparable with those in humans undergoing surgical procedures, and no teratogenic effects were observed in rats or rabbits [20,35,36].

Human epidemiologic studies have been carried out since the early 1970s to assess the potential risks of occupational exposure to the halogenated agents. Like the nitrous oxide studies, many of these studies were retrospective, mailed questionnaire surveys. They inquired about previous reproductive outcomes, for which validation was not available, and no exposure data were available. Because of the era, many of the studies predated the introduction of desflurane, sevoflurane, and modern scavenging systems. The early studies with halothane and isoflurane showed an increase in spontaneous abortions in exposed female anesthesiologists and nonphysician female operating room personnel [21–24,26]. However, later studies failed to show that exposure to anesthetic agents caused an increased risk of spontaneous abortion [27–29,37].

A more recent meta-analysis that excluded the more methodologically flawed studies estimated the relative risk of spontaneous abortion in unscavenged environments to be 1.9 (95% confidence interval, 1.72–2.09) [38]. Another recent study of the effects of working in the presence of unscavenged anesthetic gases was published in the veterinary medicine literature in 2008. This survey of Australian veterinarians showed a significant increase in the risk of spontaneous abortion in women exposed to at least 1 hour per week of unscavenged anesthetic gases [39]. Another study of female veterinarians in 2009 reported an increased rate of preterm deliveries in veterinarians who worked with unscavenged anesthetic gases [40].

As for the risk of congenital anomalies, there is less evidence for an association with occupational exposure to halogenated anesthetic agents. A few early studies reported a risk [23,26,41], but other subsequent studies reported no association with congenital anomalies [25,27,28].

There is little evidence for risk or safety of the newer, commonly used inhalational anesthetics desflurane and sevoflurane. In general, they are considered in the same manner as isoflurane. They all have National Institute for Occupational Safety and Health recommendations for a maximum exposure of 2 parts per million. Studies have shown that sevoflurane concentrations during inhaled inductions frequently exceed this limit even in the presence of properly functioning modern scavenging systems [42]. In pediatric anesthesiologists, who perform significantly more inhalational inductions than their nonpediatric anesthesiologist colleagues, a higher prevalence of spontaneous abortions has been observed [43].

Despite questions about design issues or selection bias in some studies, and the lack of evidence for the newer inhalational agents, the weight of the evidence regarding potential risks from exposure to anesthetic agents in unscavenged environments warrants concern. Scavenging is now routine, and the stance of the ASA is that there is no association between occupational exposure to trace levels of anesthetic gases in properly scavenged operating rooms and adverse health effects in pregnant women. It is still important to be aware of the risks, and practitioners need to take responsibility for ensuring a low-leakage anesthesia machine, high room ventilation rates, a functioning scavenging system, no intermittent mask ventilation, low gas flows, and control of the amount of leakage around an endotracheal tube, laryngeal mask airway, or bag-mask airway. These measures, in conjunction with working in an environment that has a properly functioning, modern scavenging system, can help ensure that the exposure levels are as low as possible. Exposure badges to measure the levels of nitrous oxide and halogenated agents are available if one is interested in measuring their level of exposure.

Radiation

Whether it is intraoperative fluoroscopy for orthopedic or intravascular procedures, or radiation from providing anesthesia in off-site locations such as the computed tomography (CT) scanner or interventional radiology suites, radiation exposure has become more and more common for anesthesiologists. Radiation can certainly cause harm to a developing fetus, so it is an important topic to address for pregnant anesthesia providers.

Ionizing radiation transfers energy to atoms and molecules, causing them to become ionized or excited. This process produces free radicals, breaks chemical bonds, produces new chemical bonds and cross-linkages, and ultimately damages the molecules (DNA, RNA, and proteins) that regulate vital cell processes. Cells do have the ability to repair a certain level of damage. However, when higher levels of damage occur, the cells cannot repair themselves and cell death occurs. With high levels of cellular death, the cells cannot be replaced quickly enough, and the involved tissues fail to function.

The sensitivity to radiation of specific tissues is proportional to the rate of proliferation of its cells, and inversely proportional to the degree of cellular differentiation. Because a developing fetus initially has a high percentage of poorly differentiated cells and a high rate of cellular proliferation, in utero exposure to ionizing radiation carries significant risk. Outcomes that have been associated with in utero ionizing radiation exposure include miscarriage, growth restriction, microcephaly, mental retardation, organ malformation, and the later development of childhood cancers, such as leukemia [44–47]. The risks are dose dependent, and seem to be highest during weeks 8 to 25 of gestation.

Several units are used when discussing radiation exposure. The traditional unit of absorbed dose is the rad, and 1 rad is equal to 100 erg/g. In the International System, the SI unit is known as the gray, and 1 Gy is equal to 1 J/kg. The conversion between these 2 units of energy and mass is 1 Gy = 100 rad. The dose equivalent is obtained by multiplying the absorbed dose (rad or gray) by a quality factor (Q) related to the damaging ability of the type of radiation. The dose equivalent units are the traditional rem (roentgen equivalent in man) and the International System sievert (Sv), and 1 Sv = 100 rem.

Radiation risk by dose has been studied, and the United States Nuclear Regulatory Commission has established occupational dose limits for declared pregnant women [47]. The annual total occupational radiation dose limit for adults is 5000 mrem (50 mSv), and the limit for total radiation exposure throughout pregnancy is 500 mrem (5 mSv), with a monthly equivalent dose limit of 50 mrem (0.5 mSv). Although these are the limits, the goal is to minimize radiation and keep exposure as low as reasonably achievable (ALARA) throughout pregnancy.

The exposure limits are based on the established radiation risks at different doses [47] (Table 1). For prenatal exposures of less than 500 mrem, there are no indications from scientific studies that harm to the fetus can result. Between 500 mrem and 5000 mrem (the occupational limit for adult radiation workers), there have been no observable effects on fetal growth or development. However, there is an increased risk of the later development of childhood leukemia and other cancers in those who were exposed prenatally. At exposures of 5000 mrem to 50,000 mrem, there are increased risks of miscarriage, mental retardation and other central nervous system abnormalities (as low as 10,000–25,000 mrem exposures), and the later development of cancers. At very high levels of radiation exposure, 50,000 to 100,000 mrem, as seen with an atomic bomb, there are risks of miscarriage, neonatal death, severe mental retardation, microcephaly, and the later development of cancers.

There are indisputable risks of radiation exposure to pregnant women, but how much radiation is one exposed to as an anesthesiologist? This exposure varies by practice setting, and the dose received depends on the duration of exposure, distance from the source, and degree of shielding. In 1 anesthesiology department the mean radiation exposure doubled in the 6 months after the introduction of a new electrophysiology service [48]. Anesthesiologists in

Table 1
Risk associated with varying levels of prenatal radiation exposure

Exposure level	Associated risks
<500 mrem	No indication of harm
500–5000 mrem	Offspring develop childhood leukemia, other childhood cancers
5000–50,000 mrem	Miscarriage, mental retardation, central nervous system abnormalities, offspring develop childhood cancers
>50,000 mrem	Miscarriage, neonatal deaths, severe mental retardation, microcephaly, central nervous system abnormalities, childhood cancers

Annual total occupational radiation dose limit for adults: 5000 mrem
Total throughout pregnancy radiation dose limit: 500 mrem
Monthly radiation dose limit in pregnancy: 50 mrem

this group increased their average exposure to almost 500 mrem per year, the occupational limit for a pregnant provider.

Several references are available and several studies have been carried out to determine the average dose of radiation received by an individual having various radiographic studies [49–51]. Single radiographs typically expose the patient to less than 1 mSv, whereas CT scans involve exposures of 5 to 12 mSv. Interventional radiology, cardiac catheterization, and angiography procedures can result in exposures up to 20 to 70 mSv. These are the exposure levels for the patient receiving a single procedure, and not the occupational exposure of the health care provider.

Occupational exposure levels have also been studied, and as expected, the exposure to the health care providers is significantly less than it is for the patient [48,52–54]. However, providers are repeatedly exposed to these lower levels, and the dose of radiation is cumulative. When considering cardiac catheterization laboratory procedures, which are typically among the highest radiation procedures performed, the occupational radiation exposure for cardiologists ranged from 0.2 to 38 μSv in 1 meta-analysis [55]. This finding shows that even the highest radiation procedures have low levels of exposure for the health care providers. These exposures are orders of magnitude less than the total pregnancy limit of 5 mSv, and the monthly limit of 0.5 mSv. However, it is conceivable that these limits could be reached if pregnant anesthesia providers were repeatedly working in these higher radiation environments throughout their pregnancies. For other health care workers, a study from 2001 using conservative values estimated that fetal dose limits might be exceeded in pregnant cardiologists after just 34 cardiac catheterization procedures, and after 87 procedures for pregnant catheterization laboratory nurses. Fig. 1 [54] is a graphic representation of unshielded, occupational radiation exposure levels compared with the monthly limit during pregnancy. These high levels do not necessarily represent the fetal exposure levels, because the measurements are obtained from unshielded parts of the body. However, this figure does show the significant amount of radiation present in these environments.

Another source of significant radiation is radiotherapy. In some institutions, anesthesia providers are asked to provide anesthesia for patients receiving radiotherapy to kill cancer cells. The amount of radiation delivered to the patient in this setting is often on the order of 20 to 60 Sv. This amount exceeds the total pregnancy limit (5 mSv), as well as the annual total occupational radiation dose limit for adults (50 mSv). Because of these high levels of radiation, these procedures are carried out in specialized settings where all health care providers leave the room and monitor the patient by cameras while the radiation is delivered. Nuclear medicine procedures using the radionucleotide technetium 99 m involve radiation doses of 1 to 7 mSv, and should also be avoided by pregnant personnel.

Although the principle of ALARA is the goal with radiation exposure, it cannot be expected that radiation exposure during pregnancy is zero. Because

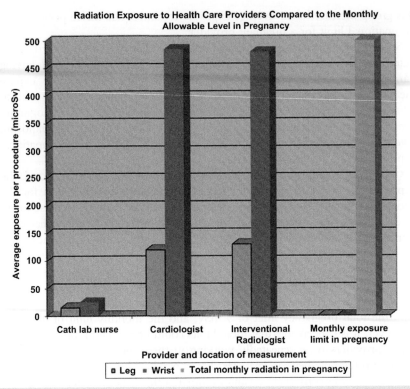

Radiation Exposure to Health Care Providers Compared to the Monthly Allowable Level in Pregnancy

Fig. 1. The average radiation exposure per procedure, as measured from the unshielded wrists and legs of various health care providers, is depicted along with the total monthly exposure limit pregnancy (500 μSv).

of this situation, it is important to have an understanding of radiation safety. The 3 basic principles of radiation safety are time, distance, and shielding. Time is straightforward; one strives to limit the total exposure time as much as possible. For distance, the dose of radiation is inversely proportional to the square of the distance from the source. So if you triple your distance from the source of radiation, your exposure is one-ninth what it was. It is recommended that health care providers stand back 1.8 m (6 ft) from the source of radiation to minimize their exposure, and further than that does not significantly decrease the exposure because the decrease is asymptotic. Radiation exposure can be further decreased by the use of shields. These shields can be lead aprons or lead panels that are placed between the radiation source and the anesthesiologist. The standard lead aprons have either 0.4-mm or 0.5-mm lead equivalence ratings. On average, they allow 8% and 3.2% transmission of a direct beam of radiation from 101.5 cm (40 in) away. Pregnancy lead aprons that have an extra-abdominal panel are available, and have a 1.0-mm lead equivalence to further decrease the amount of transmitted radiation. The lead panels come in a variety of thicknesses from 0.5 to 1.0 mm, and can be positioned between the anesthesiologist and the source of radiation to aid in shielding.

Ionizing radiation can cause fetal harm, and exposure should be limited during pregnancy. Exposure can be limited by avoiding higher-dose radiation procedures, limiting duration of exposure, positioning oneself 1.8 m (6 ft) from the radiation source, and using appropriate shielding. Radiation exposure can also be monitored with the use of dosimetry badges, which may involve wearing 1 badge on the outside collar of the lead apron and another over the abdomen under the lead apron. This method allows monitoring of the total dose of radiation exposure and the dose that the fetus could be exposed to under the lead. A radiation safety officer should be designated at all locations that use radiation, and this person should be available to answer questions related to safety during pregnancy.

MRI

MRI does not involve ionizing radiation. It works through powerful magnetic fields that align the magnetization of atoms; applied intermittent radiofrequency fields then alter the alignment of this magnetization. The nuclei of the cells produce a rotating (flipping) magnetic field that is detectable by the MRI scanner. This information is recorded and used to construct an image. Because of the physics of MRI scanning, there could be an increased risk of developmental abnormalities and teratologic effects. The developing brain may be particularly susceptible to the effects of movement-induced currents, because orientation effects are important for guiding growth of neuronal dendrites. However, there is no clinical evidence of fetal harm from in utero exposure to MRI.

MRI has been used to evaluate obstetric, placental, and fetal abnormalities for 25 years, but there are few studies concerning the relative safety of MRI in pregnant patients. In vitro studies on proliferating human cells have shown no adverse effects of static and time-varying magnetic fields [56]. Animal studies on the safety of fetal exposure to MRI have not been conclusive, and although there are design flaws with the studies, there is some evidence that fetal MR exposure may cause reduced intrauterine growth in rats and mice [57,58]. However, human studies have not revealed any adverse fetal outcomes from in utero exposure to MRI [59–63]. Specifically, there has been no reduction in fetal growth, no increase in disease or disability, and no hearing loss in the children postnatally. So at this point there are no known biologic effects to a developing fetus, but no long-term studies have been documented. The position of the American College of Radiology (ACR) is that MRI may be used in pregnant women if other nonionizing forms of imaging are inadequate, or if the examination provides information that would otherwise have required exposure to ionizing radiation. The ACR states that pregnant patients should be informed that, to date, there has been no indication that the use of clinical MRI during pregnancy has produced deleterious effects.

There is even less information about the possible effects of occupational exposure to MRI. A survey of 280 pregnant MRI professionals by Kanal and colleagues [64] showed no increase in adverse outcomes, such as sponta-neous abortions, conception taking longer than 12 months, delivery at less than 39 weeks, and birth weight less than 2.5 kg (5.5 pounds). The ACR Guideline Document for Safe MR Practices from 2007 states that pregnant health care practitioners are permitted to work in and around the MR environment throughout all stages of their pregnancy. Although they are permitted to work in the MR environment, the ACR requests that pregnant health care practitioners do not remain within the MR scanner during data acquisition or scanning [65]. This procedure may or may not require a limitation on the practice of a pregnant anesthesia provider, because there are differences in the way in which anesthetized patients are monitored during MRI scans.

Medications and chemicals

In the environments in which they commonly work, anesthesiologists are exposed to numerous medications and chemicals. Some of these substances can be hazardous to a developing fetus. Although it may not be a fully inclusive list, the agents listed in Table 2 may pose some risk to the pregnant anesthesia provider [66–68].

Inhaled medications

There are inhaled medications that anesthesia providers may be exposed to when working with particular patient populations. Often these medications are not administered in the operating room, but may be given in an intensive care unit. The 2 most common inhaled medications that pose risks to pregnant health care providers are pentamidine and ribavirin.

Pentamidine is an inhaled agent used in the treatment of *Pneumocystis carinii* pneumonia. It has been shown to be both teratogenic and embryolethal in animal studies [69,70]. In a human study of health care workers at 2 different institutions, exposure levels were calculated to be 9.8 mg/kg/d and 1.7 mg/kg/d forthose working with aerosolized pentamidine [71] Based on animal data for embryolethality and teratogenicity, these levels are greater than the embryole-thal reference dose (0.08 mg/kg/d), and near the teratogenic reference dose

Table 2
Medications, chemicals, and infections to avoid during pregnancy

Medications and chemicals to be avoided	Medications and chemicals that require care in handling
Pentamidine	Mycophenolate
Ribavirin	Cyclophosphamide
Organic solvents (ethylene oxide)	Methotrexate
Methylmethacrylate (avoid excessive inhalation)	Fluorouracil
Collodion (avoid excessive inhalation)	Mitomycin
Infectious patients to avoid if the pregnant provider is not immune	
Fifth disease	
Varicella and herpes zoster	

(4 mg/kg/d). Because of the risk of fetal harm, and the levels that providers may be exposed to, pregnant practitioners should not care for patients during the administration of aerosolized pentamidine.

Ribavirin is an inhaled medication used most commonly for the treatment of respiratory syncytial virus. It is delivered via a small-particle aerosol generator for optimum distribution in the airways. Small doses of ribavirin have been shown to cause birth defects in laboratory animals, but it is not known whether they can cause similar effects in humans [72–74]. During the administration of aerosolized ribavirin health care providers are exposed to some degree. Based on the teratogenic effects seen in animal studies, it is recommended that pregnant women avoid exposure to aerosolized ribavirin.

Intravenous medications

Anesthesiologists prepare, handle, administer, and dispose of intravenous medications on a daily basis. Depending on the type of practice, especially if it involves a surgical transplant service, one may come in contact with medications that could pose a risk to pregnant providers. Antirejection and antineoplastic agents, by way of their mechanisms of action, can be teratogenic and embryolethal. Because of this situation, particular care in handling should be taken, using full barrier precautions to avoid skin and mucous membrane contact, ingestion, or inhalation.

Mycophenolate, or Cellcept, is a noncompetitive, reversible inhibitor of inosine monophosphate dehydrogenase (IMDPH). IMDPH inhibition causes depletion of guanine nucleotide derivatives. Because they are dependent on the de novo pathway for purine biosynthesis, lymphocyte proliferation is inhibited. This situation is beneficial to help prevent rejection in transplant surgeries, but fetal exposure can have teratogenic effects. In rats and rabbits, mycophenolate has been shown to be teratogenic, and in human case reports, it seems to be as well [75–77]. Among 14 infants who were exposed to mycophenolate in utero, 12 had microtia, 9 had external auditory canal atresia, 7 had orofacial clefts, and 6 had cardiovascular malformations. There are no reports of adverse outcomes in health care workers who have had occupational exposure to mycophenolate, but providers should be aware of the risks associated with the medications they handle.

Cyclophosphamide is an antineoplastic and immunosuppressive agent that may be encountered in the operating room. It is a known teratogen, and much research has been undertaken to try to understand the multiple mechanisms by which damage occurs. Cyclophosphamide is a nitrogen mustard alkylating agent that adds an alkyl group to the guanine base of DNA. This process results in the formation of DNA cross-links between and within DNA strands, leading to cell death and disruption of the integrity of the genome. Cyclophosphamide also disrupts the embryonic epigenome and the functionality of the proteome, and these perturbations are related to teratogenesis. Cyclophosphamide induces cell-cycle arrest and apoptosis in the embryo. Clinically, the primary fetal defects that are seen are central nervous system and skeletal anomalies in rats, mice, rabbits, monkeys, and humans [78–81]. Again, there are no reports of birth defects in the offspring of occupationally exposed health care providers, but it is important to have an understanding of the risk associated with these medications.

Methotrexate is another agent that anesthesiologists may come in contact with. It is an antimetabolite, antifolate drug that inhibits the metabolism of folic acid and the synthesis of DNA, RNA, and proteins. It is used to terminate pregnancies in the early stages, so it is embryolethal, especially early in gestation. Throughout pregnancy, methotrexate also shows significant teratogenicity, with skull and limb abnormalities being seen most frequently in humans [82–84]. Care should be taken when handling this agent, and all of the embryolethal and teratogenic medications, so that self-contamination is avoided by health care providers.

Other medications

Fluorouracil and mitomycin are 2 medications that may be encountered during ophthalmic surgeries. Fluorouracil is a pyrimidine analogue antimetabolite that is commonly administered as a chemotherapeutic agent. It works through noncompetitive inhibition of thymidylate synthase to block the synthesis of thymidine, a nucleotide required for DNA replication. Because it interferes with DNA replication, fetal development can be affected if there is in utero exposure. Mice, rats, and hamsters exposed to fluorouracil during gestation had an increase in fetal resorptions and malformations such as cleft palates, skeletal defects, and deformed appendages, paws, and tails [85–88]. There are no adequate and well-controlled studies with fluorouracil in pregnant humans, but it is rated as pregnancy category D. Although most anesthesiologists do not administer chemotherapy, exposure to fluorouracil may come from ophthalmologists in the operating room who use this medication to reduce fibroblastic proliferation and subsequent scarring. This procedure helps augment trabeculotomy during glaucoma surgery to improve results.

Mitomycin is another agent that may be used by ophthalmologists during glaucoma surgery or laser eye surgery to prevent scarring and haze. It is primarily an alkylating chemotherapeutic agent that cross-links DNA and inhibits DNA synthesis. It is a pregnancy category D medication, and animal studies have revealed evidence of teratogenicity [89–91]. But again, there are no controlled studies in human pregnancy. In clinical practice, it often comes as a powder that is reconstituted in the operating room before injection by the ophthalmologist. Exposure during reconstitution and drug delivery could occur if one is not careful to avoid self-contamination. Because mitomycin interferes with DNA synthesis, exposure of a pregnant provider could result in fetal risks.

Methylmethacrylate

Methylmethacrylate is a commonly used compound for cementing total joint replacements. It has a distinctive odor that can be smelled even when it is significantly less than what is considered to be the hazardous level. Animal studies have been conflicting, but some have shown that inhalational exposure can cause an increase in fetal resorptions, birth defects, low birth weights, and delayed ossification when pregnant rats are exposed [92–94]. Documented human studies are lacking, but the US Environmental Protection Agency states that chronically exposed pregnant women had "complications during pregnancy." The doses and duration of exposure are not specified, and the types of complications are not described. Based on the evidence that exists, the Occupational Safety and Health Administration (OSHA) has set the permissible exposure limit at 100 parts per million, and methlymethacrylate is classified as pregnancy risk category C. This classification means that either studies in animals have revealed adverse effects in the fetus but no controlled studies have been reported, or studies in women and animals are not available. So the risk is unclear, but may exist if pregnant providers are exposed to the vapors of methylmethacrylate.

Collodion

Collodion is an adhesive agent that is used by some surgeons to obtain a watertight seal after certain types of skin closures. An example of its clinical use is by urologists to reinforce the closure after a scrotal orchiopexy. The major components of collodion are 60% to 70% diethyl ether, which gives it its characteristic odor, and 20% to 25% ethyl alcohol. As might be expected based on its components, collodion has been shown to be both teratogenic and mutagenic in animal studies [95]. When inhaled in poorly ventilated areas, it has anesthetic effects because of the diethyl ether, and can cause dizziness, drowsiness, unconsciousness, respiratory failure, and even death. Because of its human risks, OSHA has set occupational inhalational limits of 400 parts per million for ethyl ether, and 1000 parts per million for ethyl alcohol. No particular limits exist for pregnant workers, but because fetal risk may exist, it seems prudent to limit the exposure of pregnant women to collodion.

Organic solvents

A final group of chemicals that anesthesiologists may come in contact with in the operating room are the organic solvents. Although anesthesiologists tend not to handle these chemicals directly, they may be exposed when others in the operating room are using them. Ethylene oxide is a solvent that can be used for sterilizing surgical instruments. In pregnant laboratory animals, ethylene oxide has been shown to increase malformations and fetal loss [96–98]. In humans, exposure during pregnancy has been shown to increase the risk of spontaneous abortions [99–102]. One study reported the relative risk to be 2.5 for spontaneous abortion, and 2.7 for preterm birth [102]. OSHA recognizes this risk, and its standards for ethylene oxide require monitoring of workers' exposure, health surveillance, and provision of personal protective equipment. Respiratory protection is part of this standard, and special consideration should be given to workers whose facial features change during pregnancy.

Children whose mothers were exposed to other organic solvents, such as those in floor and tile cleaners, glues, laboratory reagents, paint thinners, paint removers, and aerosol sprays, have been shown to have higher rates of major malformations, spontaneous abortions, and visual deficits. These children have also been shown to have poorer performance with regard to neurocognitive function, language, and behavior measures [103,104]. Although anesthesiologists do not commonly use these chemicals, pregnant providers should be aware of the hazards that may exist if they are around someone who is using such products (eg, to strip or clean the floors in the operating rooms).

Infectious patients

Anesthesiologists regularly care for patients with communicable diseases. It is important for everyone to practice universal precautions to limit their risk of contracting such diseases as hepatitis and human immunodeficiency virus infection. However, pregnant providers also need to be aware of a few additional diseases that pose particular threats during pregnancy [105].

Fifth disease is a mild viral illness caused by human parvovirus B19. It often starts with mild fever, sore throat, and flulike symptoms. A classic slapped-cheeks red rash develops in most children, along with a lacy or bumpy rash on the body, arms, and legs. The virus is spread through contact with secretions of the nose and lungs, and through contact with blood. Pregnant women who do not have immunity from previous fifth disease infection have a 20% to 30% risk of infection following exposure. If a nonimmune woman contracts the disease in the first 20 weeks of gestation, there is about a 10% risk of fetal loss. Infection after 20 weeks of gestation has a risk of fetal loss of about 1%. In addition to the risk of fetal loss, there is also a risk of fetal infection. Fetal infection with fifth disease can lead to myocarditis and anemia. If the heart damage or anemia is severe, fetal hydrops can occur and may lead to fetal or neonatal death [106–113].

If there is concern for fifth disease infection in a pregnant woman, the obstetrician should be consulted. Blood tests for IgM and IgG can be performed, and serial ultrasound examinations are performed to evaluate the fetus for signs of hydrops. Depending on the gestational age, signs of fetal hydrops may be an indication for early delivery. Because infection with fifth disease can cause grave fetal harm, nonimmune pregnant providers should avoid contact with patients who have fifth disease, and always practice good hand washing.

Varicella and herpes zoster are common infections that can be risky for pregnant women who do not have immunity. Offspring of nonimmune pregnant women who contract varicella or zoster have a risk of congenital varicella syndrome. Congenital varicella syndrome includes scars on the skin, muscle and bone defects, malformed limbs, vision problems, and mental retardation. The risk of such birth defects is approximately 2%, and is highest in the first 20 weeks of gestation [114–118]. Late in pregnancy, if chickenpox develops a few days before delivery, the baby may be born with a potentially life-threatening infection. Immune globulin usually reduces the severity of the illness, and antiviral drugs may also be used. Because there are significant known risks, it is advisable for nonimmune pregnant women to avoid contact with those who have varicella or zoster infection. Pregnant women who are immune from a previous infection are not at risk and can safely care for patients with varicella or zoster infection.

In 2009 the novel H1N1 influenza virus received a lot of attention. Pregnant women experienced more severe disease, were more likely to be hospitalized, had more intensive care unit admissions, and had a disproportionately higher risk of mortality [119–121]. Early antiviral treatment appeared to be associated with fewer admissions to an intensive care unit and fewer deaths, but the best treatment was prevention through vaccination and avoidance of disease exposure. Although H1N1 is not a current issue for pregnant anesthesia providers, it shows that new risks can arise. As they arise, they need to be investigated and the possible occupational risks to the pregnant anesthesia provider should be considered.

SUMMARY

For the pregnant anesthesia provider there are many potential occupational hazards. These hazards include the inhaled anesthetics we work with every day, the ionizing radiation we are frequently exposed to, MRI that some work in proximity to, the medications and chemicals we handle, and the infectious patients we come in contact with. Education aids in identifying the risks, understanding the types of exposures, and realizing the degree of risk associated with various levels of exposure.

The risks associated with waste anesthetic gases can be minimized by ensuring that there is a properly functioning, modern scavenging system, a low-leakage anesthesia machine, high room ventilation rates, no intermittent mask ventilation, low gas flows, and adequate control of the amount of leakage around an endotracheal tube, laryngeal mask airway, or bag-mask airway. Radiation exposure can be minimized through limiting duration of exposure, maximizing distance from the source, and using proper shielding. The risks of MRI are unclear, and the current recommendations state that pregnant personnel should not remain in the scanner room during scanning. The medications and chemicals that may pose a risk should be avoided or handled with gloves and proper personal protective equipment as appropriate to each medication. Patients with certain infections that may be harmful to nonimmune pregnant providers are best avoided if a nonpregnant colleague can care for them.

Although risks exist, education brings understanding, and understanding brings the realization that there are simple ways to protect oneself so that pregnant anesthesia providers can safely continue to work throughout their pregnancies.

References

[1] FREIDA Online (database of the American Medical Association). Available at: www.freida.ama-assn.org/. 2009. Accessed March 6, 2011.

[2] American Association of Nurse Anesthetists. Available at: www.aana.com/. Accessed March 6, 2011.

[3] Regan L, Rai R. Epidemiology and the medical causes of miscarriage. Baillière's Best Pract Res Clin Obstet Gynaecol 2000;14:839–54.

[4] Martin JA, Hamilton BE, Sutton PD, et al. Are preterm births on the decline in the United States? Recent data from the national vital statistics system. National vital statistics reports; no 39. Hyattsville (MD): National Center for Health Statistics; 2010.

[5] Bird TM, Hobbs CA, Cleves MA, et al. National rates of birth defects among hospitalized newborns. Birth Defects Res A Clin Mol Teratol 2006;76(11):762–9.

[6] Ad hoc committee on effects of trace anesthetic agents on health of operating room personnel: waste anesthetic gases in operating room air: a suggested program to reduce personnel exposure. Park Ridge (IL): American Society of Anesthesiologists; 1981.

[7] McGregor DG, Baden JM, Bannister C, et al. Task Force on Trace Anesthetic Gases of the ASA committee on occupational health: waste anesthetic gases: information for management in anesthetizing areas and the postanesthesia care unit. Park Ridge (IL): American Society of Anesthesiologists; 1999.

[8] Nunn JF. Clinical aspects of the interaction between nitrous oxide and vitamin B12. Br J Anaesth 1987;59:3–13.

[9] Hansen DK, Billings RE. Effects of nitrous oxide on macromolecular content and DNA synthesis in rat embryos. J Pharmacol Exp Ther 1986;238:985–9.

[10] Deacon R, Lumb M, Perry J, et al. Selective inactivation of vitamin B12 in rats by nitrous oxide. Lancet 1978;2:1023–4.

[11] Amess JAL, Burman JF, Rees GM, et al. Megaloblastic erythropoiesis in patients receiving nitrous oxide. Lancet 1978;2:339–42.

[12] Nunn JF, Sharer NM, Gorchein A, et al. Megaloblastic erythropoiesis after multiple short-term exposure to nitrous oxide. Lancet 1982;1:1379.

[13] Fink BR, Shepard TH, Blandau RJ. Teratogenic activity of nitrous oxide. Nature 1967;214:146–8.

[14] Mazze RI, Wilson AI, Rice SA, et al. Reproduction and fetal development in rats exposed to nitrous oxide. Teratology 1984;30(2):259–65.

[15] Viera E, Cleaton-Jones P, Austin JC, et al. Effects of low concentrations of nitrous oxide on rat fetuses. Anesth Analg 1980;59:175–7.

[16] Smith BE, Gaub ML, Moya F. Teratogenic effects of anesthetic agents: nitrous oxide. Anesth Analg 1965;44:726–32.

[17] Corbett TH, Cornell RG, Endres JL, et al. Effects of low concentrations of nitrous oxide on rat pregnancy. Anesthesiology 1973;39:299–301.

[18] Mazze RI, Wilson AL, Rice SA, et al. Reproduction and fetal development in mice chronically exposed to nitrous oxide. Teratology 1982;26(1):11–6.

[19] Mazze RI, Fujinaga M, Rice SA, et al. Reproductive and teratogenic effects of nitrous oxide, fentanyl and their combination in Sprague-Dawley rats. Br J Anaesth 1987;59(10):1291–7.

[20] Fujinaga M, Baden JM, Yhap EO, et al. Reproductive and teratogenic effects of nitrous oxide, isoflurane, and their combination in Sprague-Dawley rats. Anesthesiology 1987;67(6):960–4.

[21] Cohen EN, Belville JW, Brown BW. Anesthesia, pregnancy and miscarriage. A study of operating room nurses and anesthetists. Anesthesiology 1971;35:343–7.

[22] Knill-Jones RP, Moir DD, Rodrigues LV, et al. Anaesthetic practice and pregnancy: Controlled survey of women anaesthetists in the United Kingdom. Lancet 1972;1:1326–8.

[23] American Society of Anesthesiologists: occupational disease among operating room personnel: a national study. Anesthesiology 1974;41:321–40.

[24] Rosenberg P, Kirves A. Miscarriages among operating theatre staff. Acta Anaesthesiol Scand Suppl 1973;53:37–42.

[25] Cohen EN, Brown BW, Wu ML, et al. Occupational disease in dentistry and chronic exposure to trace anesthetic gases. J Am Dent Assoc 1980;101:21–31.

[26] Pharoah PO. Outcome of pregnancy among women in anaesthetic practice. Lancet 1977;1:34–6.

[27] Rosenberg PH, Vanttinnen H. Occupational hazards to reproduction and health in anaesthetists and paediatricians. Acta Anaesthesiol Scand 1978;22:202–7.

[28] Axelsson G, Rylander R. Exposure to anaesthetic gases and spontaneous abortion: response bias in a postal questionnaire study. Int J Epidemiol 1982;11:250–6.

[29] Tannenbaum TN, Goldberg RJ. Exposure to anesthetic gases and reproductive outcome. J Occup Med 1985;27:659–68.

[30] Rowland AS, Baird DD, Weinberg CR, et al. Reduced fertility among women employed as dental assistants exposed to high levels of nitrous oxide. N Engl J Med 1992;327:993–7.

[31] Rowland AS, Baird DD, Shore DL, et al. Nitrous oxide and spontaneous abortion in female dental assistants. Am J Epidemiol 1995;141:531–8.

[32] Basford AB, Fink BR. The teratogenicity of halothane in the rat. Anesthesiology 1968;29:1167–73.

[33] Wharton RS, Wilson AI, Mazze RI, et al. Fetal morphology in mice exposed to halothane. Anesthesiology 1979;51:532–7.

[34] Mazze RI, Wilson AI, Rice SA, et al. Fetal development in mice exposed to isoflurane. Teratology 1985;32(3):339–45.

[35] Kennedy GL, Smith SH, Keplinger ML, et al. Reproductive and teratologic studies with isoflurane. Drug Chem Toxicol 1977;1:75–88.

[36] Mazze RI, Fujinaga M, Rice SA, et al. Reproductive and teratogenic effects of nitrous oxide, halothane, isoflurane, and enflurane in Sprague-Dawley rat. Anesthesiology 1986;64:339–44.

[37] Buring JE, Hennekens CH, Mayrent SL, et al. Health experiences of operating room personnel. Anesthesiology 1985;62:325–30.

[38] Bolvin JF. Risk of spontaneous abortion in women occupationally exposed to anaesthetic gases: a meta-analysis. Occup Environ Med 1997;54:541–8.

[39] Shirangi A, Fritschi L, Holman CDJ. Maternal occupational exposures and risk of spontaneous abortion in veterinary practice. Occup Environ Med 2008;65:719–25.

[40] Shirangi A, Fritschi L, Holman CDJ. Associations of unscavenged anesthetic gases and long working hours with preterm delivery in female veterinarians. Obstet Gynecol 2009;113:1008–17.

[41] Corbett TH, Cornell RG, Endres JL, et al. Birth defects among children of nurse anesthetists. Anesthesiology 1974;41:341–4.

[42] Hoerauf KH, Wallner T, Akca O, et al. Exposure to sevoflurane and nitrous oxide during four different methods of anesthetic induction. Anesth Analg 1999;88(4):925.

[43] Gauger VT, Voepel-Lewis T, Rubin P, et al. A survey of obstetric complications and pregnancy outcomes in paediatric and nonpaediatric anaesthesiologists. Pediatric Anesthesia 2003;13(6):490–5.

[44] International Commission of Radiological Protection. Recommendations of the ICRP Publication 60. Oxford (United Kingdom): Pergamon Press; 1991.

[45] International Commission on Radiological Protection, Pregnancy and Medical Radiation. Annals of the ICRP Publication 84. Oxford (United Kingdom): Pergamon Press; 2000.

[46] Wagner L, Fabrikant J, Fry R, et al. Radiation bioeffects and management text and syllabus. Am Coll Radiol 1991;164.

[47] Instruction concerning prenatal radiation exposure, regulatory guide 8.13, Revision 3. Washington, DC: United States Nuclear Regulatory Commission; 1999.

[48] Katz JD. Radiation exposure to anesthesia personnel: the impact of an electrophysiology laboratory. Anesth Analg 2005;101:1725–6.

[49] Wagner LK, Lester RG, Saldana LR. Prenatal risks from ionizing radiations, ultrasound, magnetic fields and radiofrequency waves. In: Exposure of the patient to diagnostic radiations: a guide to medical management. 2nd edition. Madison (WI): Medical Physics Publishing; 1997. p. 77–105.

[50] Toppenberg K, Hill DA, Miller DP, et al. Safety of radiographic imaging during pregnancy. Am Fam Physician 1999;59(7):1813–8.

[51] McCollough C, Schueler BA, Atwell TD, et al. Radiation exposure and pregnancy: when should we be concerned? Radiographics 2007;27(4):909–17.

[52] Kicken PJH, Kemerink GJ, van Engelshoven JMA. Dosimetry of occupationally exposed persons in diagnostic and interventional arteriography (part I: assessment of entrance doses). Radiat Prot Dosim 1999;82:93–103.

[53] McParland BJ, Nosil J, Burry B. A survey of the radiation exposures received by the staff at two cardiac catheterization laboratories. Br J Radiol 1990;63:885–8.

[54] Osei EK, Kotre CJ. Equivalent dose to the fetus from occupational exposure of pregnant staff in diagnostic radiology. Br J Radiol 2001;74:629–37.

[55] Kim KP, Miller DL, Balter S, et al. Occupational radiation doses to operators performing cardiac catheterization procedures. Health Phys 2008;94(3):211–27.

[56] Supino R, Bottone MG, Pellicciari C, et al. Sinusoidal 50 Hz magnetic fields do not affect structural morphology and proliferation of human cells in vitro. Histol Histopathol 2001;16:719–26.

[57] Mevissen M, Buntenkotter S, Loscher W. Effects of static and time-varying (50 Hz) magnetic fields on reproduction and fetal development in rats. Teratology 1994;50:229–37.

[58] Heinrichs WL, Fong P, Flannery M, et al. Midgestational exposure of pregnant BALB/c mice to magnetic resonance imaging conditions. Magn Reson Imaging 1988;6:305–13.

[59] Kok RD, de Vries MM, Heerschap A, et al. Absence of harmful effects of magnetic resonance exposure at 1.5 T in utero during the third trimester of pregnancy: a follow-up study. Magn Reson Imaging 2004;22(6):851–4.

[60] Baker PN, Johnson IR, Harvey PR, et al. A three-year follow-up of children imaged in utero with echo-planar magnetic resonance. Am J Obstet Gynecol 1994;170:32–3.

[61] Myers C, Duncan KR, Gowland PA, et al. Failure to detect intrauterine growth restriction following in utero exposure to MRI. Br J Radiol 1998;71:549–51.

[62] Clements H, Duncan KR, Fielding K, et al. Infants exposed to MRI in utero have a normal paediatric assessment at 9 months of age. Br J Radiol 2000;73:190–4.

[63] Reeves MJ, Brandreth M, Whitby EH, et al. Neonatal cochlear function: measurement after exposure to acoustic noise during in utero MR imaging. Radiology 2010;257(3):802–9.

[64] Kanal E, Gillen J, Evans JA, et al. Survey of reproductive health among female MR workers. Radiology 1993;187:395–9.

[65] Kanal E, Barkovich AJ, Bell C. ACR Guidance Document for Safe MR Practices: 2007. AJR Am J Roentgenol 2007;188:1–27.

[66] NIOSH alert: preventing occupational exposure to antineoplastic and other hazardous drugs in health care settings. Atlanta (GA): National Institute for Occupational Safety and Health; 2004.

[67] Reproductive hazards of handling medications. Pharmacist's Letter/Prescriber's Letter 2006;22:220339.

[68] Timpe E, Motl SE, Hogan ML. Environmental exposure of health care workers to category D and X medications. Am J Health Syst Pharm 2004;61(15):1556–7.

[69] Harstad TW, Little BB, Bawdon RE, et al. Embryofetal effects of pentamidine isethionate administered to pregnant Sprague-Dawley rats. Am J Obstet Gynecol 1990;163:912–6.

[70] Little BB, Harstad TH, Bawdon RE, et al. Pharmacokinetics of pentamidine in Sprague-Dawley rats in late pregnancy. Am J Obstet Gynecol 1991;164:927–30.

[71] Ito S, Koren G. Estimation of fetal risk from aerosolized pentamidine in pregnant health-care workers. Chest 1994;106(5):1460–2.

[72] Arnold SD, Alonso R. Ribavirin aerosol: methods for reducing employee exposure. AAOHN J 1993;41(8):382–92.

[73] Ito S, Koren G. Exposure of pregnant women to ribavirin-contaminated air: risk assessment and recommendations. Pediatr Infect Dis J 1993;12(1):2–5.

[74] Harrison R. Reproductive risk assessment with occupational exposure to ribavirin aerosol. Pediatr Infect Dis J 1990;9(Suppl 9):S102–5.

[75] Klieger-Grossmann C, Chitayat D, Lavign S, et al. Prenatal exposure to mycophenolate mofetil: an updated estimate. J Obstet Gynaecol Can 2010;32(8):794–7.

[76] Perez-Aytes A, Ledo A, Boso V, et al. In utero exposure to mycophenolate mofetil: a characteristic phenotype? Am J Med Genet A 2008;146(1):1–7.

[77] Anderka MT, Lin AE, Abuelo DN, et al. Reviewing the evidence for mycophenolate mofetil as a new teratogen: case report and review of the literature. Am J Med Genet A 2009;149(6):1241–8.

[78] Ozolins TR. Cyclophosphamide and the Teratology Society: an awkward marriage. Birth Defects Res B Dev Reprod Toxicol 2010;89(4):289–99.

[79] Heringová L, Jelínek R, Dostál M. Cell-cycle alterations underlie cyclophosphamide-induced teratogenesis in the chick embryo. Birth Defects Res A Clin Mol Teratol 2003;67(6):438–43.

[80] Kola I, Folb PI, Parker MI. Maternal administration of cyclophosphamide induces chromosomal aberrations and inhibits cell number, histone synthesis, and DNA synthesis in preimplantation mouse embryos. Teratog Carcinog Mutagen 1986;6(2):115–27.

[81] Mirkes PE. Cyclophosphamide teratogenesis: a review. Teratog Carcinog Mutagen 1985;5(2):75–88.

[82] Lloyd ME, Carr M, McElhatton P, et al. The effects of methotrexate on pregnancy, fertility and lactation. QJM 1999;92(10):551–63.

[83] Lewden B, Vial T, Elefant E, et al. Low dose methotrexate in the first trimester of pregnancy: results of a French collaborative study. J Rheumatol 2004;31(12):2360–5.

[84] Martínez Lopez JA, Loza E, Carmona L. Systematic review on the safety of methotrexate in rheumatoid arthritis regarding the reproductive system (fertility, pregnancy, and breastfeeding). Clin Exp Rheumatol 2009;27(4):678–84.

[85] Grafton TF, Bazare JJ Jr, Hansen DK, et al. The in vitro embryotoxicity of 5-fluorouracil in rat embryos. Teratology 1987;36(3):371–7.

[86] Wilson JG, Jordan RL, Schumacher H. Potentiation of the teratogenic effects of 5-fluorouracil by natural pyrimidines I. Biological aspects. Teratology 1969;2(2):91–7.

[87] Online reference. Available at: www.druglib.com/druginfo/fluorouracil. Accessed March 23, 2011.

[88] Abraham LM, Selva D, Casson R, et al. The clinical applications of fluorouracil in ophthalmic practice. Drugs 2007;67(2):237–55.

[89] Abraham LM, Selva D, Casson R, et al. Mitomycin: clinical applications in ophthalmic practice. Drugs 2006;66(3):321–40.

[90] Inouye M, Kajiwara Y. Teratogenic interactions between methylmercury and mitomycin-C in mice. Arch Toxicol 1988;61(3):192–219.

[91] Seller MJ, Perkins KJ. Effect of mitomycin C on the neural tube defects of the curly-tail mouse. Teratology 1986;33(3):305–9.

[92] Singh AR, Lawrence WH, Autian J. Embryonic-fetal toxicity and teratogenic effects of a group of methacrylate esters in rats. J Dent Res 1972;51:1632.

[93] McLaughlin RE, Reger SI, Barkalow JA, et al. Methylmethacrylate: a study of teratogenicity and fetal toxicity of the vapor in the mouse. J Bone Joint Surg Am 1978;60:355–8.

[94] Solomon HM, McLaughlin JE, Swenson RE, et al. Methyl methacrylate: inhalation developmental toxicity study in rats. Teratol 1993;48(2):115–25.

[95] Collodion, U.S.P. Material safety data sheet. 222 Red School Lane. Phillipsburg (NJ): Mallinckrodt Baker, Inc 08865; 2006.

[96] Generoso WM, Rutledge JC, Cain KT, et al. Exposure of female mice to ethylene oxide within hours after mating leads to fetal malformation and death. Mutat Res 1987;176(2):269–74.

[97] LaBorde JB, Kimmel CA. The teratogenicity of ethylene oxide administered intravenously to mice. Toxicol Appl Pharmacol 1980;56:16–22.

[98] Polifka JE, Rutledge JC, Kimmel GL, et al. Exposure to ethylene oxide during the early zygotic period induces skeletal anomalies in mouse fetuses. Teratology 1996;53(1): 1–9.

[99] Hemminki K, Mutanen P, Saloniemi I, et al. Spontaneous abortions in hospital staff engaged in sterilising instruments with chemical agents. Br Med J (Clin Res Ed) 1982;285(20):1461–3.

[100] Gresie-Brusin DF, Kielkowski D, Baker A, et al. Occupational exposure to ethylene oxide during pregnancy and association with adverse reproductive outcomes. Int Arch Occup Environ Health 2007;80(7):559–65.

[101] Olsen G, Lucas L, Teta J. Ethylene oxide exposure and risk of spontaneous abortion, preterm birth, and postterm birth. Epidemiology 1997;8(4):465–6.

[102] Rowland AS, Baird DD, Shore DL, et al. Ethylene oxide exposure may increase the risk of spontaneous abortion, preterm birth, and postterm birth. Epidemiology 1996;7(4): 363–8.

[103] Laslo-Baker D, Barrera M, Knittel-Keren D, et al. Child neurodevelopmental outcome and maternal exposure to solvents. Arch Pediatr Adolesc Med 2004;158(10):956–61.

[104] Julvez J, Grandjean P. Neurodevelopmental toxicity risks due to occupational exposure to industrial chemicals during pregnancy. Ind Health 2009;47(5):459–68.

[105] Hood J. The pregnant health care worker–an evidence-based approach to job assignment and reassignment. AAOHN J 2008;56(8):329–33.

[106] Anderson LG. Human parvovirus B19. Pediat Ann 1990;19(9):509–13.

[107] Chisaka H, Ito K, Niikura H, et al. Clinical manifestations and outcomes of parvovirus B19 infection during pregnancy in Japan. Tohoku J Exp Med 2006;209(4):277–83.

[108] Gillespie SM, Cartter ML, Asch S, et al. Occupational risk of human parvovirus B19 infection for school and daycare personnel during an outbreak of erythema infectiosum. JAMA 1990;263:2061–5.

[109] Jordan JA. Placental cellular immune response in women infected with human parvovirus B19 during pregnancy. Clin Diagn Lab Immunol 2001;8(2):288–92.

[110] Kailasam C. Congenital parvovirus B19 infection; experience of a recent epidemic. Fetal Diagn Ther 2001;16(1):18–22.

[111] Sailer DN, Rogers BB, Canick A. Maternal serum biochemical markers in pregnancies with fetal parvovirus B19 infection. Prenat Diagn 1993;12(6):467–741.

[112] Soulie JC. Cardiac involvement in fetal parvovirus B19 infection. Pathol Biol Paris 1995;43(5):416–9 [in French].

[113] Tolfvenstam T, Broliden K. 2009. Parvovirus B19 infection. Semin Fetal Neonatal Med 2009;14(4):218–21.

[114] Pastuszak AL, Levy M, Schick B, et al. Outcome after maternal varicella infection in the first 20 weeks of pregnancy. N Engl J Med 1994;331(7):482.

[115] Chapman SJ. Varicella in pregnancy. Semin Perinatol 1998;22:339–46.

[116] Enders G, Miller E, Cradock-Watson J, et al. Consequences of varicella and herpes zoster un pregnancy: prospective study of 1739 cases. Lancet 1994;343:1547.

[117] Koren G. Congenital varicella syndrome in the third trimester. Lancet 2005;366: 1591–2.

[118] Jones KL, Johnson KA, Chambers CD. Offspring of women infected with varicella during pregnancy: a prospective study. Teratology 1994;49(1):29–32.

[119] Siston AM, Rasmussen SA, Honein MA, et al. Pandemic 2009 influenza A(H1N1) virus illness among pregnant women in the United States. JAMA 2010;303(15): 1517–25.

[120] Louie JK, Acosta M, Jamieson DJ, et al. Severe 2009 H1N1 influenza in pregnant and postpartum women in California. N Engl J Med 2010;362(1):27–35.

[121] ANZIC Influenza Investigators Australasian Maternity Outcomes Surveillance System. Critical illness due to 2009 A/H1N1 influenza in pregnant and postpartum women: population based cohort study. BMJ 2010;340:c1279.

Advances in Anesthesia 29 (2011) 59–84

ADVANCES IN ANESTHESIA

Veterinary Anesthesia

Carrie A. Schroeder, DVM*, Lesley J. Smith, DVM

Department of Surgical Sciences, School of Veterinary Medicine, University of Wisconsin, 2015 Linden Drive, Madison, WI 53706, USA

W hereas the practice of veterinary medicine is centuries old, veterinary anesthesia is relatively young, originating in the mid-nineteenth century [1]. At that time, chloroform was the dominant agent used to induce an anesthetic state in veterinary patients, although agents such as ethyl chloride, chloral hydrate, and cyclopropane were also used [1]. The widespread practice of veterinary anesthesia began in the 1920s with the discovery of the barbiturates, and pentobarbitone was the first to be widely used [1]. Prior to the acceptance of this pharmacologic means of restraint, anesthesia and analgesia of animals involved far more physical than chemical restraint. Over the years and decades that followed, veterinary anesthesia continued to evolve, accepting the use of halogenated anesthetics, opioids, nitrous oxide, and tranquilizers. As the art and science of general anesthesia evolved in veterinary medicine, it became clear that specialization of veterinarians in anesthesia was necessary. In 1964, a group of scientists and veterinarians with a shared interest in anesthesia founded the Association of Veterinary Anaesthetists in Europe, but no certification in this specialty was offered. In the late 1960s and early 1970s, the charter members of the American College of Veterinary Anesthesiologists (ACVA) worked closely with physician anesthesiologists to establish formal training programs in veterinary anesthesia. After a great deal of work by these charter members, the ACVA was founded in 1975. The European counterpart of the ACVA is the European College of Veterinary Anaesthesia and Analgesia (ECVAA), founded in 1995. Both of these organizations serve to certify veterinarians specializing in veterinary anesthesia through residency programs and subsequent certification examinations.

Today, the majority of anesthesia of veterinary species is practiced in private clinics by veterinary technicians and veterinarians not specialized in veterinary anesthesia. In the United States, there are currently more than 61,000 veterinarians working on domestic, food and fiber, performance, and exotic species

The authors have nothing to disclose.

*Corresponding author. 1109 Observatory Hill Drive, Belleville, WI 53509. E-mail address: carada@uwalumni.com

0737-6146/11/$ – see front matter
doi:10.1016/j.aan.2011.07.002

in private practices; most of these practitioners perform and oversee anesthesia without additional postgraduate training [2]. Although the exact rates of anesthetic-related morbidity and mortality in veterinary clinics is not known, a study of small animal clinics in the United Kingdom revealed the risk of anesthetic and sedation-related death of healthy dogs and cats (American Society of Anesthesiologists [ASA] status 1–2) to be 0.05% and 0.11%, respectively. These rates are in stark contrast to human perioperative mortality rates, reported to be less than 0.001% for surgical inpatients [3]. These statistics are more remarkable when one considers that the vast majority of dogs and cats presenting to veterinarians are young ASA 1–2 patients requiring general anesthesia for elective ovario-hysterectomy or castration, as compared with the human population that usually requires general anesthesia because of underlying disease, congenital abnormalities, or injury. Mortality rates in veterinary medicine increase to 1.33% and 1.40% for dogs and cats, respectively, determined to be systemically ill (ASA status 3–5) [4].

The rates of perioperative mortality are much higher for other species, approximately 2% to 4% in small rodents and up to 16% in small birds [4]. A similar study of perioperative fatality of horses in the United Kingdom revealed an overall mortality rate of 1.9% [5]. Horses presenting for emergency surgery had a much higher mortality rate, reported to be approximately 4 to 9 times higher depending on the required procedure [6].

There are multiple factors that may account for these differences in anesthetic-related mortality between veterinary and human medicine. Such factors include the lack of adequate patient history and presenting complaints, as animals cannot communicate their medical complaints and veterinarians must rely on history (as reported by owners); physical examination; and other diagnostics to infer medical conditions. These many aspects highlight the need for thorough physical examination and often lead veterinarians to recommend preanesthetic diagnostics such as thoracic radiographs, serum chemistry, and complete blood counts as basic health-screening tools. These diagnostics may help to reveal occult medical problems that may not be evident on physical examination or to the animal's owner. Another potential factor accounting for the difference in perioperative mortality may be financial constraints of veterinary practices, including the cost of more advanced anesthetic monitoring equipment, the cost of a well-stocked pharmacy allowing for individualization of anesthetic plans, and the cost of a dedicated veterinarian or veterinary technician to monitor anesthesia. In the case of exotic small patients and horses, there are additional reasons to postulate why these species have increased anesthetic-related mortality, including body size, difficulty in monitoring, species-specific stress responses, and in the case of horses, mortality associated with difficulties in anesthetic recovery. Because of their strong flight response, horses will often panic if they are not able to stand easily after anesthesia, or may attempt to stand before they are fully recovered from the central nervous system (CNS) effects of anesthetics. Manual assistance of horses in recovery is often performed, but is potentially dangerous to personnel.

In addition to these factors, the lack of advanced training in anesthesia may account for some difference in the overall mortality rates. At present, there are only 220 veterinarians in the United States who are diplomats of the ACVA. While many veterinarians are well experienced in anesthesia, the additional training and expertise of board-certified individuals could help decrease the overall morbidity and mortality rates of domestic and exotic animal species.

The training of veterinary anesthesiologists is similar to that of physician anesthesiologists. Following 4 years of veterinary school, 1 year of practice experience or internship unrelated to anesthesia is required. Following this prerequisite, a 3-year residency under the supervision of diplomats of the ACVA is required. At present there are 20 residency programs registered with the ACVA in the United States. The standard training program incorporates anesthesia of multiple species with multiple disease processes, the practice of advanced techniques such as regional anesthesia, and completion of a research project resulting in publication. Following completion of the residency program, a written examination of the ACVA must be passed followed by the successful completion of an oral examination.

The field of veterinary anesthesia is similar to the human field, not only in the certification process; the equipment, drugs, and anesthetic techniques used share many similarities with those of human anesthesia. There are, however, key differences in tailoring anesthetic techniques to patients ranging in size from mice to whales, including species' temperament and natural behavior, logistics, body size, human safety, available equipment and drugs, and patient medical status.

EQUIPMENT

The myriad of shapes, sizes, and physiologic differences presented by veterinary species presents several challenges regarding anesthetic equipment.

Anesthetic delivery systems

In veterinary anesthesia, anesthetic delivery systems must be available in a wide range of sizes to deliver volatile anesthetics and ventilate very small and very large patients. For the majority of cases, the anesthesia machines used for veterinary anesthesia are similar to those designed to deliver volatile anesthetics to humans. It is not a requirement for anesthesia machines used on veterinary species to comply with guidelines set by the American Society for Testing and Materials (ASTM), therefore some of the machines used in veterinary practice may be considered obsolete by some standards. However, these machines have often been either refurbished or updated to deliver modern anesthetics with precision and safety. In most veterinary practices, precision out-of-circuit vaporizers are used, but older styles of vaporizers such as the copper kettle may be found in some practices.

Most inhalational anesthesia in veterinary clinics is performed on companion animals, specifically dogs and cats. Breeds of dogs can range in size from less than 1 kg (eg, a chihuahua puppy) to greater than 100 kg (eg, an adult mastiff).

Cats are more uniform in size, typically weighing 4 to 5 kg, with kittens weighing approximately 0.5 to 1 kg. Pediatric or adult rebreathing (circle) systems are used in patients weighing more than 3 kg. Patients weighing less than 3 kg generally require non-rebreathing systems for anesthetic delivery [7]. Exotic species, such as small birds or hamsters, often weighing less than 100 g, may be mask-induced and then maintained on non-rebreathing systems. Specialized piston-driven ventilators have been developed to provide positive-pressure ventilation to these small species. The MicroVent ventilator developed by Hallowell EMC (Fig. 1) allows veterinarians to deliver intermittent positive-pressure ventilation and high-frequency oscillatory ventilation to small patients, with tidal volumes ranging from 0 to 10 mL.

At the other end of the spectrum are domestic and exotic large animals. Horses and cattle are typically maintained under general anesthesia with volatile anesthetics delivered via specialized large animal anesthetic circle systems, machines, and ventilators (Fig. 2). With an average horse weighing approximately 500 kg, and light and heavy breeds weighing anywhere from 300 to 1000 kg, large animal rebreathing circuits with an inner diameter of 50 mm are coupled with either a 30-L rebreathing bag or 18-L ventilator bellows. For extremely large animals requiring inhalant anesthesia, specialized anesthesia delivery equipment has been developed. An example of this is the elephant ventilator designed by Mallard Medical, Inc (Figs. 3 and 4). This ventilator was designed for patients up to 9 tons, delivering a tidal volume up to 125 L at a flow rate of 1100 L/min. It uses two large animal ventilators and circuits connected in parallel. Field ventilation of this enormous species has

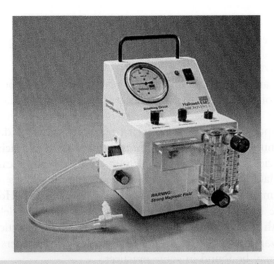

Fig. 1. The Hallowell EMC MicroVent 1, a specialized ventilator designed to provide intermittent positive-pressure ventilation or high-frequency oscillatory ventilation to extremely small veterinary patients. (*Courtesy of* Hallowell EMC, Pittsfield, MA; with permission.)

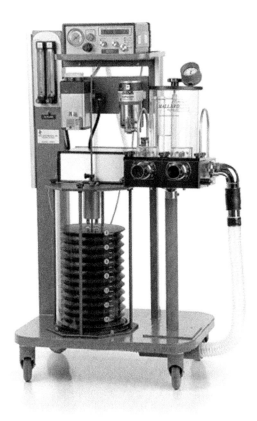

Fig. 2. Large animal ventilator designed for use on species heavier than 100 kg. Features include 18-L ascending bellows and flowmeters providing fresh gas flow ranging from 0 to 10 L/min. (*Courtesy of* Mallard Medical Inc, Redding, CA; with permission.)

also been described using a similar modification of two high-flow demand valves [8]. Administration of positive-pressure ventilation using this technique improved P_aO_2 in one elephant from 40 to 366 mm Hg [8].

Airway devices

In comparison with humans, the laryngeal structures and tracheae of dogs are very large. Large breeds of dogs can easily accommodate an endotracheal tube with an inner diameter (i.d.) of 12 to 14 mm. Small to medium-sized breeds are typically intubated with endotracheal tubes ranging in size from 5 to 9 mm i.d. Cats typically accommodate endotracheal tubes ranging in size from 3.5 to 4.5 mm i.d. Moderately sized birds and reptiles are intubated using commercially available endotracheal tubes with 2 to 2.5 mm i.d. Considerably smaller birds and reptiles need a more creative approach; a size 16 to 18 standard wire gauge (SWG) intravascular catheter can be easily adapted to attach to the anesthetic

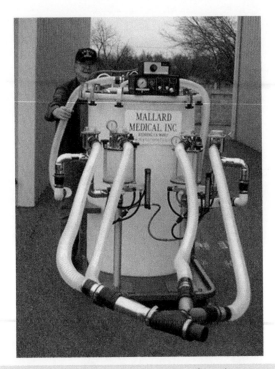

Fig. 3. Elephant ventilator designed by the connection of two large animal ventilators in parallel. This ventilator was designed to provide positive-pressure ventilation for patients weighing up to 9 tons and is capable of delivering tidal volumes up to 125 L. (*Courtesy of* Mallard Medical Inc, Redding, CA; with permission.)

circuit by removing the stylet and inserting the adaptor from a 3-mm i.d. endotracheal tube. Specialized endotracheal tubes are commercially available for large animals; a horse or cow is typically intubated with a 24- to 30-mm i.d. endotracheal tube. Endotracheal tubes of considerably larger size have been developed, and are used for megavertebrate species such as elephants and giraffes.

Veterinary laryngoscopes are adapted from human laryngoscopes. Miller and McIntosh blades are most common. A small McIntosh blade is well suited for cats and small primates, and a large Miller blade, up to 205 mm, is suitable for large dogs. Specialized Miller-style blades designed for pigs and ruminants, such as cattle and goats, are typically 350 to 450 mm in length.

The use of laryngeal mask airways (LMAs) has been reported in dogs, cats, rabbits, pigs, and primates [9–13]. However, because of large patient size variations and the relative ease in which most of these species are intubated, LMAs are not extensively used in veterinary anesthesia.

General anesthesia can be induced in small exotic species with volatile anesthetics delivered via facemasks. However, some species and individual patients

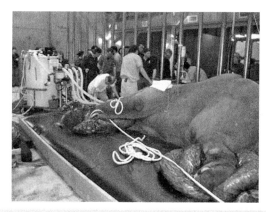

Fig. 4. Ventilation of a 7-ton Asian elephant at the Portland Zoo. (*Courtesy of Mallard Medical Inc, Redding, CA; with permission.*)

that cannot be adequately restrained for intravenous catheterization or inhalational induction via facemask can be successfully anesthetized by means of an anesthetic induction chamber (Fig. 5). These chambers can be purchased commercially or manufactured by modifying a glass aquarium to seal and accept either a fresh gas inlet or both inspiratory and expiratory limbs of the anesthetic circuit. This means of anesthetic induction is slow because of the relatively large volume of the anesthetic chamber, creates a large amount of environmental contamination, and is typically stressful to the patient. Therefore, volatile anesthetic administration via chamber is generally reserved for situations whereby there is no alternative means of delivery.

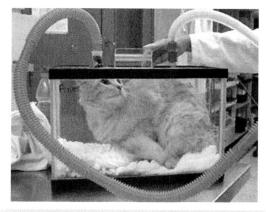

Fig. 5. Anesthetic induction chamber used for administration of volatile anesthetics to a fractious cat.

Anesthetic monitors

Anesthetic monitors are like those used in human anesthesia. Many private veterinary practices minimally monitor their patients with a pulse oximeter, while a noninvasive blood pressure monitor is also often implemented. Extremes of size and heart rate (ranging from 25 beats/min in horses to >300 beats/min in birds) can make measurement of blood pressure by oscillometric means difficult, as many of these monitors lose accuracy at these extremes. The application of a small Doppler ultrasound crystal to amplify peripheral pulse sounds can be coupled with a sphygmomanometer to obtain noninvasive arterial blood pressure for species in which blood pressure measurement via oscillometry is less accurate. In more critical patients and when available skill allows, veterinary patients may be monitored with invasive blood pressure techniques.

Pulse oximeter probes designed for use on the human finger can be clamped across an animal's tongue but, once again, extremes of size limit the utility of this modality. Flat reflectance probes can be placed over the palantine artery, in the proximal esophagus, or the rectum if use of a transmittance probe is unsuccessful. This technique is often used in small exotic species, but veterinarians must take the class of the animal into account. Commercially available pulse oximeters are designed for use on the mammalian oxygen-hemoglobin dissociation curve. Measurements obtained from the pulse oximeter placed on other classes of animals such as birds or reptiles may not be accurate.

Electrocardiography (ECG) monitoring is implemented in many veterinary practices. A 3-lead system is often used, either with alligator-style clips attached to the skin or ECG patches placed on the footpads or shaved spots on the body. ECG clips can be adapted to very small patients such as birds by attaching alligator clips to 25-SWG needles passed through the skin. The ECG waveform is reasonably well conserved across species. One notable difference is the prominent Ta wave (representing atrial repolarization) seen in horses, producing the appearance of a bifid p wave.

DRUGS

As is the theme for much of veterinary anesthesia, the drugs used by veterinarians to sedate and anesthetize animals are very similar to the drugs chosen by physicians for this purpose. However, there are some key drugs that are not shared in common by the two professions. Some of the drugs used today have been developed specifically for veterinary use, whereas others are drugs that were originally developed for use in humans and have found a niche in the veterinary market. However, most of these drugs are not specifically labeled for the species in which they are used, which is a common hurdle in veterinary medicine, but veterinarians are protected by the Animal Medicinal Drug Use Clarification Act, which permits extralabel ("off-label" to the human anesthesiologist) drug use by veterinarians. One reason that many anesthetic drugs are not approved by the Food and Drug Administration (FDA) for use in animals is the expense incurred by pharmaceutical companies in obtaining FDA approval in light of a limited veterinary market.

Veterinarians administering drugs to food-animal species such as pigs, chickens, and cattle need to be aware of the specific meat or dairy withdrawal times of the drugs they are using, a factor of utmost importance in preventing potentially toxic drugs from entering into the food chain. To address this potential complication, the United States Department of Agriculture sponsors the Food-Animal Residue Avoidance and Depletion program, which maintains a database of the appropriate timing in which drugs can be given before slaughter or collection of milk.

Much like pediatric sedation, many veterinary species require sedation with sedative or neuroleptic drugs before anesthetic induction agents can be administered. While some animals require only mild to moderate sedation, drugs that provide complete chemical restraint are occasionally needed in fractious or dangerous species. Preanesthetic sedation is typically given via the intramuscular route, due to the greater need for physical restraint when administering drugs via the intravenous route. Following appropriate sedation patients are more cooperative, and intravenous catheterization is less stressful to the patient and veterinary staff.

There are significant species differences in the reactions to certain classes of sedative, analgesic, and anesthetic drugs. Veterinarians must be familiar with the species to avoid untoward effects.

Sedatives

Benzodiazepines are one of the drug classes in veterinary anesthesia that have significant species-specific differences in their sedative effects. However, they are widely used because they are nearly devoid of adverse cardiovascular effects, and the respiratory depression seen with this class of drugs in most species, even at high dosages, is extremely mild and well tolerated.

Diazepam is typically administered intravenously in combination with dissociative drugs to provide muscle relaxation, and its administration as a sole agent is uncommon because of the unpredictability of absorption after intramuscular injection. Midazolam is extensively used and is an excellent sedative in most small exotic species, including birds, rabbits, and ferrets. The sedation seen with most domestic species such as dogs, cats, horses, and cattle is, however, unreliable. Due to its safe cardiopulmonary side-effect profile, it is administered commonly in combination with opioids to geriatric or debilitated dogs and cats, often resulting in moderate sedation. However, the administration of midazolam to healthy domestic species often results in poor sedation, and behavioral disinhibition can occur. Well-behaved animals have been known to turn relatively unhandleable and even vicious following the sole administration of benzodiazepines.

α2 Agonists are far more reliable sedatives in most species, and are widely used. The prototypical α2 agonist is xylazine, with relatively poor specificity for the α2 receptor compared with the α1 receptor; this results in a significant amount of peripheral vasoconstriction, resulting in hypertension with a reflex bradycardia. Other α2 agonists such as detomidine, romifidine, and dexmedetomidine have been developed with improved α2:α1 specificity and improved vascular side effects. All of these agents produce significant, but reversible, sedation that is useful for preanesthetic sedation and for procedural sedation such as laceration repair and orthopedic examination. With the aid of regional anesthesia, abdominal surgery can be performed in standing large animals with sedation by α2 agonists. Paradoxically, the α2 agonists cannot be relied on for chemical immobilization in unsafe individuals or species. Horses have been known to kick on heavy xylazine sedation and apparently well-sedated dogs have been known to spontaneously rouse and bite veterinarians. However, high doses of these agents are gaining in popularity as anesthetic agents in certain exotic species. As significant cardiovascular side effects can occur, caution is needed with the indiscriminate use of these agents; significant increases in cardiac afterload can be detrimental to animals, with decreased cardiac reserve and decreases in cardiac output of 60% having been reported [14].

Phenothiazines are another commonly used class of sedatives, largely in domestic species. Acepromazine is the most widely used of this class, providing moderate sedation in most species. This class of drugs is frequently reserved for anxiolysis associated with hospitalization and preanesthetic sedation, and is often combined with opioids for greater sedation in dogs and cats. The most significant side effect of acepromazine is dose-dependent vasodilation and hypotension.

When chemical restraint is necessary for either fractious domestic species or dangerous exotic species, the dissociatives are the most reliable class of drugs in veterinary medicine. Technically speaking, this class of drugs produces chemical restraint via hypnotic effects, and not sedation, but dissociative drugs are commonly combined with other sedative preanesthetic medications. Ketamine is most frequently used but another dissociative, tiletamine, is available in combination with the benzodiazepine zolazepam in the proprietary drug Telazol (Fort Dodge Animal Health, Fort Dodge, IA). These drugs are used heavily in zoo, wildlife, and exotic animal medicine to provide chemical restraint adequate to provide safe working conditions around dangerous species such as large carnivores. Ketamine is rarely administered as a sole agent, due to excessive muscle rigidity; combination with benzodiazepines or α2 agonists is recommended. Telazol is provided as a powder that can be reconstituted with either sterile water or other anesthetic drugs to provide a highly potent anesthetic compound in a low volume, which can be easily loaded into a dart or administered intramuscularly.

Opioids are widely used in all veterinary species for analgesia and, in some species, for sedation. These drugs are often part of the premedication regimen, but are discussed in the sections that cover pain and analgesia in veterinary patients.

Induction agents

In recent times, the veterinary anesthesia community has been limited in its choices for anesthetic induction agents. The disappearance of thiopental from the United States market was a great loss for the veterinary community, leaving only 3 options for anesthetic induction: propofol, etomidate, and dissociative/benzodiazepine combinations.

Anesthetic induction of veterinary species is frequently accomplished using propofol. This drug provides a smooth anesthetic induction, adequate to provide a spectrum of anesthetic depth from titratable sedation for laceration repair to unconsciousness for endotracheal intubation. Veterinary species rarely react adversely to the intravascular injection of propofol, suggesting that the burning sensation of injection commonly reported in humans is a mild or rare occurrence in veterinary species. The 20-mL vials of propofol that are commercially available are unnecessarily large for many veterinary patients, creating the need to either share vials between patients or, because of the short shelf life, waste a large amount of the drug. A 4-kg cat, for instance, would only require approximately 20 mg, or 2 mL, of propofol, resulting in 18 mL of extra drug that needs to be used within 24 hours. Although the drug itself is not costly, the relative cost increases when such large amounts of waste are necessary. Private veterinary practices with a smaller surgical caseload may therefore avoid use of this drug for economic reasons. Recently, Abbott Animal Health has released Propoflo28, which has a reported 28-day shelf life and makes veterinary use more economical (Abbott Animal Health, North Chicago, IL). This drug does, however, contain benzyl alcohol as the solvent, which can cause hemolytic abnormalities in cats [15,16].

Dissociatives in combination with benzodiazepines are commonly used to induce a myriad of species. A combination of ketamine with diazepam is typically administered as an intravenous bolus to provide anesthetic induction. In comparison with propofol, the anesthetic induction is slower and is accompanied by a greater amount of jaw tone and laryngeal reactivity. Administration of faster-acting induction agents, such as propofol, result in rapid collapse in large animals such as a horses or cows, which could result in injury to both the animal and its handlers. The slower onset of general anesthesia provided by dissociative combinations is advantageous when inducing anesthesia in larger species, for which a more controlled induction is necessary.

Etomidate is available for use in veterinary species and is best known for the safety of its cardiovascular profile. While advantageous in animals with myocardial dysfunction, the use of this drug is often avoided because of the profound nausea and retching observed and the high cost associated with the drug. For instance, the cost of anesthetic induction of a 20-kg dog with etomidate is roughly 7 times the cost of propofol and 30 times the cost of ketamine/diazepam. This cost may prove to be unacceptably high for some veterinary practitioners.

Ultrapotent opioids are used for chemical restraint and anesthetic induction in large exotic species for capture and medical intervention. These drugs are specific to veterinary medicine. Carfentanil, approximately 10,000 times the potency of morphine, and etorphine, approximately 8000 times the potency of morphine, are the 2 most commonly used drugs in this class. These drugs allow for fast anesthetic induction with fast and nearly complete anesthetic reversal. The major advantage of this class of drugs is the small volume needed to induce anesthesia in very large species. For instance, chemical immobilization of a rhinoceros can be achieved with roughly 2 to 3 mg of etorphine, a volume as low as 0.2 to 0.3 mL. However, although the respiratory depression of the opioids is generally well tolerated in veterinary species, anesthesia with the ultrapotent opioids is characterized by significant hypoxemia. Supplemental oxygen must be administered as field conditions allow. While useful, these drugs have the potential to prove deadly to veterinarians accidentally exposed either parenterally or across mucous membranes. Purchase and use of these drugs requires a special Drug Enforcement Agency permit, and it is important for veterinarians working with this class of drugs to wear gloves and eye protection when handling the drugs, darts, and drug administration site, to prevent inadvertent exposure.

Inhalant anesthetics

The volatile anesthetics are used extensively in veterinary medicine, and their use does not differ significantly from their use in humans. Isoflurane is the most commonly used agent in veterinary practice followed by sevoflurane and, rarely, desflurane. The minimum alveolar concentration (MAC) of these agents is well conserved across species. For instance, the MAC of isoflurane and sevoflurane in the dog is approximately 1.4% and 2.4%, respectively, while in cats the MAC is 1.6% for isoflurane and 2.6% for sevoflurane [17–20].

Euthanasia solution

One of the advantages of working with veterinary species is the ability to ease an animal's suffering through euthanasia. The act of euthanasia is accomplished by intravenous injection of commercially available euthanasia solutions. Pentobarbital is the main component of these solutions, with the addition of phenytoin in certain brands. Overdose of these agents produces rapid CNS depression, cessation of respiration, and cardiovascular collapse. As agonal breathing may occur prior to death, the preadministration of propofol or high doses of sedative agents may be elected when owners are present. To prevent inadvertent administration, characteristic color dyes such as blue or pink are added for easy identification of the agent. It is important to avoid use of these agents in animals intended for use as food. Pentobarbital poisoning has been reported in Sumatran tigers following consumption of horsemeat contaminated with euthanasia solution [21].

COMPANION ANIMAL ANESTHESIA

The most common companion animals presenting for general anesthesia to veterinary practitioners are dogs and cats. However, this section also briefly summarizes some of the unique anesthetic challenges of the other companion animal species, namely horses, cattle, swine, and camelids.

Anesthetic management of these species is based on similar principles to those used in human anesthesia, whereby a balanced anesthetic approach involving multiple sedatives, analgesics, adjunctive analgesics, induction agents, and inhalants is used. The biggest challenge to the veterinary anesthetist is the differences in body size that may present within a species; for example, canine patients can range in size from 500 g to 100 kg. Another challenge is the fact that these patients are nonverbal and their behavior can be difficult to interpret, particularly during recovery.

Canine and feline anesthesia

In most canine and feline patients, intramuscular administration of sedative/ analgesic combinations are used as premedication, to reduce stress of handling, ease catheter placement, and reduce induction drug and inhalant dosage requirements. Common premedication combinations are opioids combined with benzodiazepines, acepromazine, or dexmedetomidine. Actual drug choices and doses will depend on the patient's physical status, temperament, medical history, current disease, and the procedure that is planned. In some fractious cats, ketamine or Telazol may also be coadministered to achieve chemical restraint. It is usually fairly easy to gain intravenous access via catheterization, using either the cephalic veins or the medial or lateral saphenous veins. Anesthetic induction with propofol, ketamine with diazepam, or etomidate is most common. Endotracheal intubation in the dog is performed with the animal in the prone position with the head extended, and the laryngoscope placed ventral to the epiglottis (Fig. 6). Laryngospasm in dogs is rare, so neuromuscular blocking agents are not generally used in the induction regimen. Brachycephalic breeds of dogs (eg, pugs and bulldogs) can be challenging at intubation because of their elongated soft palates, everted laryngeal saccules, and typically hypoplastic tracheas. These breeds of dogs are also at more risk for hypoxia after sedation and during recovery, due to the increased work of breathing caused by their stenotic upper airways. Supplemental oxygen and close

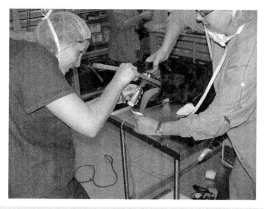

Fig. 6. Intubation of a large dog with a 12-mm internal diameter (i.d.) endotracheal tube and a Miller laryngoscope blade.

monitoring are important for these patients during these perianesthetic periods. Endotracheal intubation in cats is also easily accomplished in the same manner as for dogs; however, cats are prone to laryngospasm, which can usually be moderated by topical application of a local anesthetic such as lidocaine directly on the larynx. In dogs and cats, once intubation is accomplished, anesthetic maintenance with inhalants, and monitoring via invasive and noninvasive means is used much as in anesthesia or humans. Direct cardiac output monitoring, bispectral index monitoring, electroencephalography (EEG), cerebral blood flow, or intracranial pressure monitoring are rarely used in veterinary anesthesia, however, because of cost constraints and, in some instances (EEG), lack of data to support interpretation [22]. A challenge that veterinarians face in anesthesia of canine and feline patients is during recovery, when emergence delirium, dysphoria, and pain can be challenging to decipher. Emergence delirium can be managed by either light sedation or patient reassurance until the delirium abates. Dysphoria may be caused by opioids, particularly in Northern breeds of dogs such as malamutes and huskies. If there is also pain at recovery, however, reversal of opioids to treat the dysphoria leaves fewer options for systemic analgesia. Often the best approach in these patients is to sedate them at recovery with potent sedatives such as dexmedetomidine, but this then introduces the need for more vigilant monitoring throughout the recovery period.

Equine anesthesia

Horses that are handled often are usually amenable to intravenous catheter placement in their large jugular veins with topical or subcutaneous local anesthesia. Intravenous α2 agonists xylazine, detomidine, or romifidine, which are more cost-practical than dexmedetomidine, are commonly used for premedication. Anesthetic induction in these animals, which can weigh up to 1000 kg, presents a physical challenge. Horses have a strong flight instinct, so must be well restrained during anesthetic induction to avoid injury to themselves or personnel. Most clinics that perform general anesthesia on horses have a specialized stall or area with a squeeze gate or padded wall against which the animal is restrained during induction (Fig. 7). Intravenous induction with ketamine and diazepam or 5% guaifenesin (a centrally acting muscle relaxant) is the most common, as propofol and etomidate are cost-prohibitive, and can produce myoclonic activity and rough inductions. The animal is gently encouraged into a "dog sitting" position, eased into the prone position, then rolled into lateral recumbency and easily intubated by blind passage of a 24-mm to 30-mm i.d. endotracheal tube directly into the oropharynx with the head in extension (Fig. 8). Proper placement is confirmed by the "feel" of the tube dropping into the trachea, absence of a palpable tube in the midcervical esophagus, and expired air fogging up the lumen of the endotracheal tube. In specialized clinics and referral hospitals, many horses are then maintained on inhalants and monitored via invasive or noninvasive means, similar to anesthesia in humans. Most horses, because of their size, have a significant decrease in functional residual

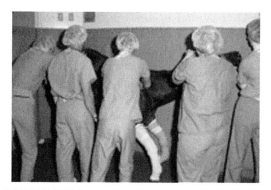

Fig. 7. Induction of general anesthesia in a horse.

capacity during recumbency, with significant ventilation-perfusion mismatch due to atelectasis and decreases in cardiac output. Therefore, many horses that are maintained under general anesthesia will suffer from significant hypercapnia and hypoxemia, despite an FiO_2 of 100%. Mechanical ventilation is common, with tidal volumes ranging from 5 to 15 L. A unique challenge in equine anesthesia is the increased risk for postanesthetic myopathy and neuropathy that can result from improper or poor padding, prolonged anesthetic times, and hypotension. Such a situation can lead to disastrous consequences during recovery, as horses will panic from inability to get to their feet from pain secondary to myopathy or from nerve damage. Risk factors should be avoided at all costs, and physical assistance of the horse during recovery via ropes on the head, attached to a halter, and tail, plus light sedation in some instances, may prevent a rough recovery or injury to the animal.

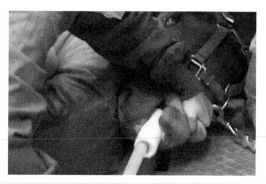

Fig. 8. Intubation of a horse with a 24-mm i.d. endotracheal tube. A polyvinylchloride pipe covered with elastic bandage material is used to keep the mouth open and protect the endotracheal tube.

In field anesthesia of the horse, which is common for simpler procedures such as castration, anesthetic induction is performed as already described, but then maintenance is accomplished by a constant rate infusion of a combination of xylazine, ketamine, and guaifenesin. Typically there is no supplemental oxygen available, padding is nonexistent, and the recumbency time should be limited to 30 minutes.

Bovine and camelid anesthesia

General anesthesia of bovids and camelids is relatively rare, due to economic constraints for farmers in pursuing extensive surgical procedures and the ease with which standing surgery can be performed in these species with sedation and regional anesthesia. When these species do require general anesthesia, an intravenous catheter can be easily placed in the jugular vein. Most cattle do not require sedation prior to induction, due to their placid temperaments. More fractious cattle, and many camelids, can be lightly sedated with low doses of xylazine (approximately 1% of the same dosage that a horse would require). After light sedation, cattle will assume a prone position, and camelids will "cush," assuming a similar position. Following anesthetic induction, with regimens like those described for horses, cattle and camelids are intubated in this position. In cattle, because of limited range of motion of their temporomandibular joint and caudally placed larynx, intubation is performed manually. A large mouth gag is used to hold the jaw open and the anesthetist inserts the endotracheal tube by physical palpation of the epiglottis and larynx, then slides the endotracheal tube past his or her hand and into the trachea (Fig. 9). Most adult cattle require a 26- to 30-mm i.d. endotracheal tube. Intubation of camelids requires a specially manufactured extra-long Miller blade laryngoscope, and a stylet is passed into the trachea as a guide over which an endotracheal tube is passed. Regurgitation during intubation in bovine and camelid species can result in significant aspiration pneumonia. For this reason, these species are usually fasted for a minimum of 24 hours before induction, but their rumen, the largest stomach compartment, can still be full of gas and fluid. Regurgitation is more common when intubation is attempted before the animal is sufficiently deep.

Swine anesthesia

General anesthesia of swine is very uncommon, with the possible exception being the pet pig or the companion Vietnamese pot-bellied pig (Fig. 10). These species are challenging to anesthetize because of numerous factors. Swine have an extremely thick layer of fat overlying muscle, so intramuscular injections must be performed with long needles (2.5–3.5 inches [6.3–8.9 cm]) to penetrate the fat layer. Pigs vocalize loudly during injection and are very difficult to restrain. A plywood board can sometimes be used to pin them against a wall or corner of a stall, but their screams are blood curdling. Sedation can be accomplished with intramuscular injection of multiple different combinations, including xylazine, ketamine, and Telazol; medetomidine and μ-agonist opioids; or, in compromised pigs, midazolam and opioids. Once the animal

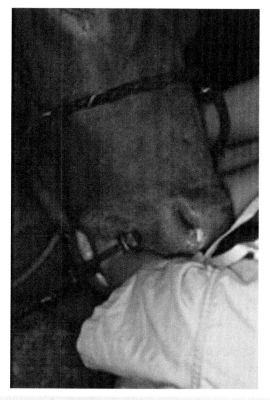

Fig. 9. Bovine intubation via manual palpation of laryngeal structures.

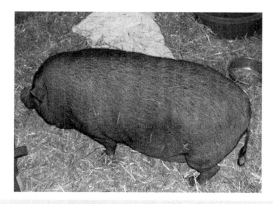

Fig. 10. A Vietnamese pot-bellied pig.

is sedated, intravenous access is also very challenging. In larger pigs, an auricular vein on the superficial surface of the ear can be easily catheterized, but in pot-bellied pigs these veins are small, tortuous, and not easy to visualize. Occasionally a cut-down approach to the cephalic vein is necessary. Induction can be with intravenous propofol or by inhalant delivered by mask if intravenous access is impossible. These species have a uniquely shaped larynx with a diverticulum on the ventral wall that acts like a blind pouch. When intubating, it is easy to get the endotracheal tube "stuck" in this pouch and it then cannot be advanced into the trachea. Rotating the endotracheal tube from concave side "down" to concave side "up" as it advances through the larynx will help to prevent obstruction in the diverticulum. These species also have very small tracheas for their body weight, so an assortment of endotracheal tube sizes should be available. Once pigs are intubated, inhalant maintenance and monitoring is similar to that for other species. Malignant hyperthermia has been reported in certain breeds of pigs, namely Pietran, Poland China, Landrace, Spotted Swine, and swine of large all white breeds, so end-tidal CO_2 and temperature monitoring is important [23]. Recovery can be very prolonged, due to the need for relatively high doses of premedications and uptake of drugs into the significant adipose tissue that continues to contribute to measureable plasma levels for hours after injection.

WILDLIFE, ZOO, AND EXOTIC ANIMAL ANESTHESIA
The art of anesthesia of nondomestic species relies on the solid knowledge and skills of domestic animal anesthesia. The physiology and anatomy of many exotic species can be analogous to domestic species. For instance, tiger anesthesia is similar, in many respects, to domestic cat anesthesia and the anesthesia of African hoofstock, such as antelope, is similar that of domestic cattle.

Anesthesia of small exotic species
Small exotic species such as birds, rodents, and rabbits are typically anesthetized using inhalational techniques. These small species may be flighty, and intravenous catheterization under manual restraint can be extremely challenging. This fact often leaves veterinary practitioners with no alternative but to induce anesthesia with volatile anesthetics using either a facemask or an induction chamber. Unfortunately, due to a lack of species-specific facemasks, this technique has the potential to result in a great deal of environmental contamination and exposure of personnel to anesthetic waste gases. In an attempt to decrease the amount of volatile anesthetic necessary and decrease anesthetic induction time, these species may be premedicated with a sedative/opioid combination.

These species are generally well sedated with midazolam, but allometric scaling is necessary, resulting in a high dose requirement. For instance, 1 to 2 mg/kg of midazolam is a reasonable dose for most small exotic species and results in moderate sedation. The partial μ agonist buprenorphine or the κ agonist butorphanol are commonly combined with midazolam, due to the synergism of sedative effects. Although pure μ agonists are effective in the small mammalian species, the potential for respiratory depression is often enough for practitioners to avoid use of these drugs, despite respiratory depression in veterinary species being generally mild and well tolerated.

Endotracheal intubation of small mammals such as guinea pigs and chinchillas is difficult, as direct visualization due to small mouth size can be challenging and these species are highly prone to regurgitation on laryngeal stimulation. Intubation of these species is rarely attempted, and anesthetic maintenance with volatile anesthetics is usually accomplished with a facemask. Rabbits, on the other hand, are simpler to intubate, either nasotracheally or orotracheally. Much like a horse, the airway of the rabbit is amenable to blind intubation when the head is placed in extension. With practice, most veterinary practitioners can readily intubate rabbits as small as 1 to 1.5 kg. Avian species can be easily intubated with direct visualization. The glottis is rostrally located and readily visible in these species, even without the aid of a laryngoscope (Fig. 11).

Anesthesia of reptiles

Because of physiologic differences that allow extended periods of apnea and the ability to shunt blood flow away from the lungs, the induction of reptiles with volatile anesthetics is often impractical and can take upwards of 10 minutes. Superficial veins are difficult to access in most reptiles, but injection of propofol into the peripheral coccygeal vein, located along the base of the vertebrae of the tail, is easily accomplished in most snakes and lizards. Anesthetic induction of chelonian species such as tortoises can be similarly accomplished using the easily accessible venous sinus located just below the shell at the base of the neck.

Like birds, reptiles can be easily intubated with direct visualization. Reptiles can even be intubated when sedated or compromised, and anesthetic induction completed with volatile anesthetics delivered through positive-pressure ventilation. Individual species may have anatomic differences that can make

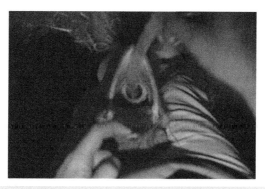

Fig. 11. Intubation of an ostrich. The neck is placed in extension, the beak opened, and the glottis readily visualized. Notice the lack of epiglottis and the rostral location of the glottis.

endotracheal intubation more difficult. For instance, crocodilians have tissue overlying the glottis and lying in apposition to the soft palate called the gular fold, which allows submerged crocodilians to rest with their mouths open without water entering the glottis. This fold is similar to a large epiglottis and can be displaced manually before intubation.

Anesthesia of large exotic species

Anesthetic induction of larger species can be accomplished by administration of chemical immobilization agents by either hand injection or remote delivery systems. Hand injections are often assisted with the aid of a squeeze cage where a movable panel is controlled by hand or pneumatics to compress the animal, restricting its movement. Remote injection can be accomplished using a pole syringe whereby the veterinarian can administer the injection by a syringe at the end of an extending device, allowing the injector to stand up to 3 m from the animal. For animals and situations whereby it is unsafe to get into close proximity, projection systems using expired air, carbon dioxide, or powdered charge can be used to propel darts containing anesthetic drugs into the animal. Several systems for darts and remote delivery are commercially available and are often tailored to the needs of the situation (Fig. 12).

Chemical immobilization of dangerous species is achieved by the combination of sedative agents either with dissociative drugs or ultrapotent opioids. These classes of drugs allow fast anesthetic induction, permitting veterinarians and wildlife biologists to perform procedures, physical examination, or physical relocation safely. When working with remote delivery systems that use darts it is important to keep in mind the volume of injectate, as excessively large patients can require multiple dart injections. For this reason, highly concentrated drugs such as Telazol or the ultrapotent opioids may be chosen. Pharmaceutics companies have developed highly concentrated forms of drugs such as medetomidine, the racemic mixture of levomedetomidine and dexmedetomidine, at 20 mg/mL.

When working with exotic animal species, it is important to administer agents and use anesthetic techniques with a fast onset to minimize stress.

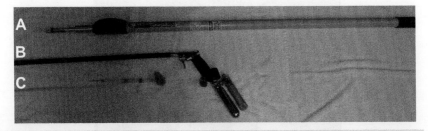

Fig. 12. Examples of equipment for remote animal capture. Displayed is a pole syringe, used for drug hand administration from approximately 1 m away (*A*), a carbon dioxide–driven pistol for propelling darts into animals (*B*), and a dart (*C*).

Nondomestic species are often, by nature, prone to extreme stress with handling, and untoward effects of this stress response can be manifested. Exertional myopathy can result when free-ranging species such as deer and other hoofstock are chased over long distances or excessively stressed. This condition can result in peracute death or renal failure from myoglobinuria.

The intubation of larger species can be accomplished either with direct laryngeal visualization, blind passage of the endotracheal tube, or manual palpation of laryngeal structures to facilitate passage of an endotracheal tube. Manual intubation of species in which placement of one's hand in the mouth is dangerous can be aided by a mouth gag to prevent mouth closure (Fig. 13).

PAIN AND ANALGESIA IN VETERINARY ANESTHESIOLOGY: A BRIEF OVERVIEW

Analgesic therapy in veterinary medicine is similar to that in human medicine, although there are significant challenges that relate to economics, species' responses to analgesic drugs, technical limitations, lack of available data on pharmacokinetics and pharmacodynamics of analgesic drugs in veterinary patients, and the fact that patient-controlled analgesia is not an option in these species. Another huge challenge in analgesic therapy is the interpretation of

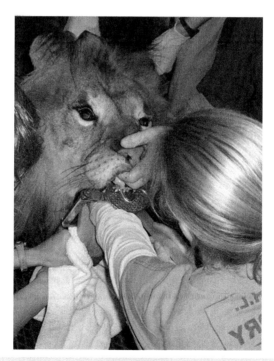

Fig. 13. Intubation of an African lion via manual palpation of laryngeal structures rather than direct visualization.

patient pain in a nonverbal animal that may respond to pain in different ways depending on instinct, learned behavior, and socialization or lack thereof. For example, prey species will "hide" signs of pain, whereas a well-socialized dog may seek company, vocalize, or otherwise draw attention to their discomfort. Behaviors related to pain can be very species specific. For example, abdominal pain in horses results in rolling, or looking at or kicking at their abdomen, violently throwing themselves against walls or to the ground, sweating, pawing, and shaking. In dogs, abdominal pain may present as depression, lethargy, in-appetance, a "hunched back" appearance, and resentment of abdominal palpa-tion. In ruminants, abdominal pain may be more difficult to detect, and the animal may simply lack interest in food, appear depressed, and grunt or grind its teeth. Cats with abdominal pain will hide, abandon grooming behavior, hiss or growl when stroked, and lose interest in food or water.

Various pain-scoring scales have been developed in veterinary medicine. A visual analog scale, similar to that used in people, can be utilized whereby the veterinarian, as opposed to the patient, puts a tick mark on a 100-mm scale reflecting where he or she interprets pain to be on a spectrum from none to unbearable. This method is clearly fraught with the potential for error and bias. Numerical rating scales have been developed that are species specific [24–26], but there is probably also a need for numerical rating scales that are specific to the type of pain expected, for example, orthopedic versus abdominal. In short, pain interpretation in veterinary medicine is in its infancy. Much of analgesic therapy is based on the expected degree of pain based on the proce-dure or disease, "instinct" in observation of the patient, and a positive patient response to analgesic treatment.

Opioids

The opioids are the mainstay of analgesia in veterinary medicine. The respira-tory depression due to opioids that is observed in most veterinary species is typically less than that observed in humans. Therefore, relatively large dosages of opioids can be used without significant untoward effects. For instance, it is not uncommon to administer 1 mg/kg of morphine intramuscularly to dogs. Mild respiratory depression may be observed, but in healthy animals is rarely of clinical significance. In one study, healthy dogs administered large doses of hydromorphone maintained $PaCO_2$ values between 43 and 48 mm Hg [27].

A potentially more significant side effect of opioids in veterinary species is CNS excitement seen in several species after μ-agonist administration, which is thought to be attributable to species differences in opioid receptor distribu-tion in the brain [28]. Horses administered high doses of μ-agonist opioids demonstrate increased locomotor activity and incoordination, a potentially dangerous side effect for both the animal and surrounding personnel [29]. The effects seen in cats are generally less dangerous, typically a euphoric state manifested as mydriasis, rolling, pawing, and kneading with the forepaws [30]. However, severe hyperthermia in cats associated with the administration of μ agonist has been documented in the literature [31]. The excitatory effects of opioids can generally be avoided by judicious use of proper dosages and coadministration with a sedative agent. It has also been observed that excitatory effects of opioids are fewer when they are administered specifically to treat existing pain, unlike when they are administered as part of a preemptive premedication combination.

Significant differences exist in the distribution and functionality of opioid receptors among species and classes of animals and, therefore, differences in the analgesic efficacy of different opioid classes exist. For instance, κ-opioid receptor agonists such as butorphanol and nalbuphine are more effective analgesics in avian species than are μ agonists [32]. The efficacy of different classes of opioids in reptile species has also been extensively studied, and analgesia in these species appears to be mediated through the μ-opioid receptor, much like mammals [33].

In veterinary medicine, opioid administration may be parenteral, epidural, spinal, or regional. The fentanyl patch is also commonly used in many species, with relatively predictable uptake and efficacy. Buprenorphine can be administered transmucosally to cats, due to the alkaline pH of cat saliva and a pKa of buprenorphine of 8.24 [34,35]. Unlike humans, most formulations of opioids that are marketed for oral administration are not useful in veterinary species, due to significant first-pass metabolism; for example, oral administration of MS Contin to dogs results in negligible serum concentrations [36]. Therefore, in the perioperative setting, veterinary patients usually receive opioids by one of the aforementioned routes, then for longer durations of analgesia are sent home with a fentanyl patch or nonopioid analgesics such as nonsteroidal anti-inflammatory drugs (NSAIDs), tramadol, or gabapentin.

NSAIDs are used commonly in veterinary medicine, and their efficacy and side-effect profile are similar to those in humans. Common NSAIDs prescribed to dogs are carprofen, ketoprofen, deracoxib, firocoxib, and meloxicam. Dosing intervals vary between the NSAIDs and renal, hepatic, and gastrointestinal side effects are common with high doses or prolonged use [37–39]. Cats are unique in that their renal prostaglandins are exquisitely sensitive to NSAIDs, and acute renal failure after NSAID use in cats is a true risk [40]. The only NSAID that is FDA-approved for use in cats is meloxicam as a one-time dose. Off-label use of NSAIDs in cats does occur, due to the valid concern for inadequate analgesic therapy with a single dose of an NSAID after major surgery, but acute renal failure may occur even in previously healthy cats. In horses, cattle, and camelids, commonly administered NSAIDs include phenylbutazone, flunixin meglumine, and firocoxib. A topical NSAID, diclofenac, is now available for use in horses, specifically for treatment of arthritis [41]. Because horses are often used as performance animals, strict rules exist by governing bodies such as the United States Equestrian Federation and the Federation Equestrienne Internationale on the use of NSAIDs and other drugs in horses used for competition purposes.

The local anesthetics are used commonly for regional or systemic analgesia in veterinary patients, particularly in dogs and horses. Epidural, spinal, and regional routes of administration are common and very effective. Cats are uniquely sensitive to the toxic effects of local anesthetics, and can develop dys-hemoglobinemias, seizure activity, and cardiovascular collapse after relatively low doses of lidocaine, bupivacaine, or benzocaine.

Other analgesic drugs, such as N-methyl-D-aspartate (NMDA) antagonists, tramadol, gabapentin, amantadine, and maropitant [42] are empirically used in veterinary medicine, with few data currently available regarding efficacy or ideal dosing intervals. Unfortunately, due to limited available funding for research in veterinary species, studies on these analgesic drugs are slow to trickle into the literature.

SUMMARY

This article provides a brief overview of some of the differences and unique challenges that veterinary anesthetists and anesthesiologists face in dealing with a myriad of veterinary patients. Species-specific differences in normal behavior, drug metabolism, CNS response to drugs, anatomy, and physiology must be considered when planning anesthetic or analgesic management of veterinary patients. Some veterinary patients can be dangerous, particularly during anesthetic induction and recovery, so personnel safety is also of concern. Differences in sheer body size means that anesthetic equipment used in veterinary medicine must be adapted or developed to meet requirements for induction, recovery, ventilatory support, and general anesthetic management. Finally, limitations in the number of board-certified veterinary anesthesiologists worldwide makes for relatively slow progress in current knowledge and published literature related to anesthetic and analgesic management of veterinary species.

References

[1] Weaver BM. The history of veterinary anesthesia. Vet Hist 1987;5(2):43–7.
[2] American Veterinary Medical Association. Market research statistics—US veterinarians. Available at: www.avma.org./reference/marketstats/usvets.asp. Accessed April 1, 2011.
[3] Li G, Warner M, Lang BH, et al. Epidemiology of anesthesia-related mortality in the United States, 1999-2005. Anesthesiology 2009;110:759–65.
[4] Brodbelt DC, Blissitt KJ, Hammond RA, et al. The risk of death: the confidential enquiry into perioperative small animal fatalities. Vet Anaesth Analg 2008;35:365–73.
[5] Johnston GM, Steffey E. Confidential enquiry into perioperative equine fatalities (CEPEF). Vet Surg 1995;24:518–9.
[6] Mee AM, Cripps PJ, Jones RS. A retrospective study of mortality associated with general anesthesia in horses: emergency procedures. Vet Rec 1998;42:307–9.
[7] Hartsfield S. Anesthetic machines and breathing systems. In: Tranquilli WJ, Thurmon JC, Grimm KA, et al, editors. Lumb & Jones' veterinary anesthesia and analgesia. 4th edition. Ames, IA: Blackwell Publishing; 2007. p. 453–94.
[8] Horne WA, Tchamba MN, Loomis MR. A simple method of providing intermittent positive-pressure ventilation to etorphine-immobilized elephants (Loxodonta africana) in the field. J Zoo Wildl Med 2001;32:519–22.
[9] Martinis RH, Braz JR, Defaveri J, et al. Effect of high laryngeal mask airway intracuff pressure on the laryngopharyngeal mucosa of dogs. Laryngoscope 2000;110:645–50.
[10] Cassu RN, Luna SP, Teixeira Neto FJ, et al. Evaluation of laryngeal mask as an alternative to endotracheal intubation in cats anesthetized under spontaneous or controlled ventilation. Vet Anaesth Analg 2004;31:213–21.

[11] Bateman L, Ludders JW, Gleed RD, et al. Comparison between facemask and laryngeal mask airway in rabbits during isoflurane anesthesia. Vet Anaesth Analg 2005;32: 280–8.

[12] Fulkerson PJ, Gustafson SB. Use of laryngeal mask airway compared to endotracheal tube with positive-pressure ventilation in anesthetized swine. Vet Anaesth Analg 2007;34: 284–8.

[13] Johnson JA, Atkins AL, Heard DJ. Application of the laryngeal mask airway for anesthesia in three chimpanzees and one gibbon. J Zoo Wildl Med 2010;41:535–7.

[14] Pypendop BH, Verstegen JP. Hemodynamic effects of medetomidine in the dog: a dose titration study. Vet Surg 1998;27:612–22.

[15] Cullison RF, Menard PD, Buck WB. Toxicosis in cats from use of benzyl alcohol in lactated Ringer's solution. J Am Vet Med Assoc 1983;182(1):61.

[16] Wilcke JR. Idiosyncrasies of drug metabolism in cats: effects of pharmacotherapeutics in feline practice. Vet Clin North Am Small Anim Pract 1984;14(6):1345–54.

[17] Steffy E, Howland D. Isoflurane potency in the dog and cat. Am J Vet Res 1984;38:1833–6.

[18] Kazama T, Ikeda K. Comparison of MAC and the rate of rise of alveolar concentration of sevoflurane with halothane and isoflurane in the dog. Anesthesiology 1988;68:435–8.

[19] Drummond JC, Todd MM, Shapiro HM. Minimal alveolar concentrations for halothane, enflurane, and isoflurane in cats. J Am Vet Med Assoc 1983;182:1099–101.

[20] Doi M, Yunoki H, Ikeda K. The minimum alveolar concentration of sevoflurane in cats. J Anesth 1988;2:113–4.

[21] Jurczynski K, Zittlau E. Pentobarbital poisoning in Sumatran tigers (Panthera tigris sumatrae). J Zoo Wildl Med 2007;38:582–4.

[22] Smith LJ, Greene SA, Moore MP, et al. Effects of arterial carbon dioxide tension on quantitative electroencephalography in halothane-anesthetized dogs. Am J Vet Res 1994;55(4): 467–71.

[23] Moon PF, Smith LJ. General anesthetic techniques in swine Anesthesia Update. Vet Clin North Am Food Anim Pract 1996;12(3):663–92.

[24] Firth AM, Haldane SL. Development of a scale to evaluate postoperative pain in dogs. J Am Vet Med Assoc 1999;214:651–9.

[25] Holton L, Reid J, Scott EM, et al. Development of a behavior based pain scale to measure acute pain in dogs. Vet Rec 2001;148:525–31.

[26] Cambridge AJ, Tobias KM, Newberry RC, et al. Subjective and objective measurement of postoperative pain in cats. J Am Vet Med Assoc 2000;217:685–9.

[27] Wunsch L, Krugner-Higby LA, Heath TD, et al. A comparison of the effects of hydromorphone HCl and a novel extended release hydromorphone on arterial blood gas values in conscious healthy dogs. Res Vet Sci 2010;88:154–8.

[28] Combie J, Dougherty J, Nugent E, et al. The pharmacology of narcotic analgesics in the horse IV. Dose and time response relationships for behavioral responses to morphine, meperidine, pentazocine, anileridine, methadone, and hydromorphone. J Equine Med Surg 1979;3:377–85.

[29] Hellyer PW, Bai L, Supon J, et al. Comparison of opioid and alpha-2 agonist adrenergic receptor binding in horse and dog brain using radioligand autoradiography. Vet Anaesth Analg 2003;30:172–82.

[30] Lascelles BD, Robertson SA. Use of thermal threshold response to evaluate the antinociceptive effects of butorphanol in cats. Am J Vet Res 2004;65(8):1085–9.

[31] Posner LP, Pavuk AA, Rokshar JL, et al. Effects of opioids and anesthetic drugs on body temperature in cats. Vet Anaesth Analg 2010;37:35–43.

[32] Paul-Murphy JR, Brunson DB, Miletic V. Analgesic effects of butorphanol and buprenorphine in conscious African grey parrots (Psittacus erithacus erithacus and Psittacus erithacus timneh). Am J Vet Res 1999;60:1218–21.

[33] Sladky KK, Miletic V, Paul-Murphy J, et al. Analgesic efficacy and respiratory effects of butorphanol and morphine in turtles. J Am Vet Med Assoc 2007;230:1356–62.

[34] Weinberg DS, Inturrisis CE, Reidenberg B, et al. Sublingual absorption of selected opioid analgesics. Clin Pharmacol Ther 1988;44:335–42.

[35] Robertson SA, Lascelles BD, Taylor PM, et al. PK-PD modeling of buprenorphine in cats: intravenous and oral transmucosal administration. J Vet Pharmacol Ther 2005;28(5):453–60.

[36] Kukanich B, Lascelles BD, Papich MG. Pharmacokinetics of morphine and plasma concentrations of morphine-6-glucuronide following morphine administration to dogs. J Vet Pharmacol Ther 2005;28(4):371–6.

[37] Jones CL, Budsberg SC. Physiologic characteristics and clinical importance of the cyclooxygenase isoforms in dogs and cats. J Am Vet Med Assoc 2000;217:721–9.

[38] Jones CL, Streppa HK, Budsberg SC. In vivo effect of a COX-2 selective and nonselective nonsteroidal anti-inflammatory drug (NSAID) on gastric mucosal and synovial fluid prostaglandin synthesis in dogs. J Vet Intern Med 2001;15:273.

[39] MacPhail CM, Lappin MR, Meyer DJ, et al. Hepatocellular toxicosis associated with administration of carprofen in 21 dogs. J Am Vet Med Assoc 1998;212:1895–901.

[40] Lascelles BD, Court MH, Hardie EM, et al. Non-steroidal anti-inflammatory drugs in cats: a review. Vet Anaesth Analg 2007;34(4):228–50.

[41] Lynn RC, Hepler DI, Kelch WJ, et al. Double-blinded placebo-controlled clinical field trial to evaluate the safety and efficacy of topically applied 1% diclofenac liposomal cream for the relief of lameness in horses. Vet Ther 2004;5(2):128–38.

[42] Gaynor JS. Other drugs used to treat pain. In: Gaynor JS, Muir WW, editors. Veterinary pain management. Saint Louis (MO): Mosby; 2002. p. 251–61.

Advances in Anesthesia 29 (2011) 85–112

ADVANCES IN ANESTHESIA

ELSEVIER
MOSBY

Perioperative Considerations and Management in Patients with Intravascular Stents

Isaac Lynch, MD[a,*], Daniel A. Emmert, MD, PhD[b],
Michael H. Wall, MD[c]

[a]Critical Care and Trauma Anesthesiology, Department of Anesthesiology, Washington
University in St Louis School of Medicine, 660 South Euclid Avenue, Campus Box 8054,
St Louis, MO 63110, USA
[b]Cardiothoracic Anesthesiology, Department of Anesthesiology, Washington University in
St Louis School of Medicine, 660 South Euclid Avenue, Campus Box 8054, St Louis,
MO 63110, USA
[c]Anesthesiology and Cardiothoracic Surgery, Department of Anesthesiology, Washington
University in St Louis School of Medicine, 660 South Euclid Avenue, Campus Box 8054,
St Louis, MO 63110, USA

OVERVIEW OF PERCUTANEOUS CORONARY INTERVENTION

There are few medical advances that have altered the landscape of their field as much as percutaneous coronary intervention (PCI). The earliest heart catheterizations were performed on animals in the eighteenth century by Hales, using metal and glass pipes [1]. Understanding of the anatomy and physiology of the heart and vascular system, as well as the nature of circulation, advanced slowly over the next century. In the late nineteenth century, Fick developed his formula for calculating cardiac output, and he and others performed animal right-heart and left-heart catheterizations. These discoveries, along with the discovery of radiographs and fluoroscopy in the late 1890s, helped pave the way for a generation of innovators who pushed the limits of medically accepted therapy.

The first pioneers of human cardiac catheterization were considered by most of their peers to be dangerous mavericks rather than revolutionaries. Werner Forssmann, who was later awarded the Nobel Prize for his work, performed the first human heart catheterization on himself (and was summarily fired) [1]. Sones, a pediatric cardiologist, developed selective coronary angiography by accident during a ventriculogram. Dotter and Judkins performed the first

The authors have nothing to disclose.

*Corresponding author. E-mail address: lynchi@anest.wustl.edu

0737-6146/11/$ – see front matter
doi:10.1016/j.aan.2011.07.003

peripheral angioplasty in 1963, when they passed an arterial catheter, by chance, through an iliac artery occlusion during an aortogram [1].

Although these initial discoveries came by happenstance, the magnitude of the event was not lost on the operators. Replicating, refining, and expanding on these early techniques, peripheral and coronary angioplasty steadily progressed until the next major advancement, the first percutaneous transluminal coronary angioplasty (PTCA) on an awake human, was performed by Andreas Gruentzig in 1977.

PTCA

After his successful procedure, Gruentzig continued to perform PTCA and published his first case series of 50 patients in 1979 [2]. The procedure gained worldwide interest, and use increased rapidly. The early equipment was cumbersome and difficult to maneuver, thereby limiting the situations in which PTCA could be implemented. The original indications were for discrete, proximal, noncalcified lesions in a single vessel [3]. Despite the crude technology, the procedure was deemed safe and effective, with an overall survival rate of 93% for single-vessel disease, and 70% of patients being free of target vessel disease at 10 years [3]. Seemingly as a testament to this fact, Gruentzig's first patient, Adolph Bachman, is still alive and with clean coronaries (Fig. 1).

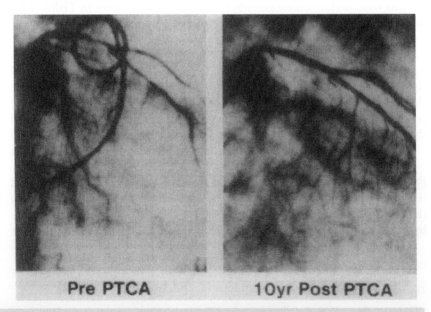

Pre PTCA   10yr Post PTCA

Fig. 1. The before and after picture of Gruentzig's first patient, Adolph Bachman. Note the circled lesion in the pre-PTCA image. (*From* Douglas JS, King SB. Hurst's the heart. McGraw-Hill, Inc., New York; 2001. p. 1437; with permission.)

After establishing the relative safety and efficacy of PTCA, researchers set about comparing it with the established therapies for coronary disease, medical management, and coronary artery bypass grafting (CABG). Meta-analyses including these early trials are skewed because the technology, operative skill, and overall safety of both PCI and CABG have increased markedly over the past 30-plus years. The early trials comparing medical management with intervention (PTCA or CABG), such as the Medicine, Angioplasty or Surgery Study (MASS) and Randomised Intervention Treatment of Angina II (RITA-II) (medical therapy vs PTCA), showed that intervention resulted in improved symptom control but a slight increase in the composite of death and myocardial infarction (MI) [4,5]. In addition, patients assigned to PTCA had an increased number of subsequent coronary interventions, including CABG. Later randomized controlled trials comparing these treatment groups, such as MASS-II, found that there is no difference in the rate of death/MI among patients assigned to medical management or intervention, and supported the findings of increased symptom relief with PTCA or CABG [6]. As seen in previous studies, need for further coronary intervention was higher in the medical management and PTCA groups. Trials comparing PTCA and CABG, such as RITA, EAST (Emory Angioplasty Versus Surgery Trial), and BARI (Bypass Angioplasty Revascularization Investigation), showed equivalent risk of death/MI, similar improvement in angina and exercise tolerance, and again an increased need for further revascularization in the PTCA group [7–9].

A closer look at the mechanism of balloon angioplasty helps to explain the trend of high rates of target vessel revascularization (TVR) after PTCA. Originally, it was the prevailing belief that balloon angioplasty was a gentle, smooth, and controlled expansion of the blood vessel, which resulted in remodeling of soft, compressible plaque and dilation of the vessel caliber. Amplatz and colleagues, in 1980, showed that the mechanism is more violent [10]. Using cadaveric and animal models, these investigators showed that dilation of the vessel causes fracturing of the plaque, disruption of the intima and media, and arterial stretching. It is an unpredictable response to sustained force on the rigid, mineralized vessel. Exposure of the plaque constituents and injury to the vessel wall explain the 2 major complications of PTCA: abrupt or acute closure and restenosis (Figs. 2 and 3).

Abrupt closure of the target vessel can be a result of acute thrombus formation at the ruptured plaque (similar to an acute MI) or vessel dissection and occlusion. It has an incidence of 3% to 5%, usually occurs within the first 24 hours of the procedure, and can lead to MI, emergency CABG, and death [11]. It was the norm to have surgical standby for PTCA, before the advent of the coronary stent [12]. Restenosis, defined as greater than 50% reduction in postprocedure lumen diameter, is the result of both elastic recoil of the smooth muscle and new growth of the injured vessel wall, termed neointimal proliferation. It usually manifests within 6 months as increasing angina, and often requires reintervention [11]. Tackling these complications became the goal of interventional cardiology, because patient safety and cost-effectiveness

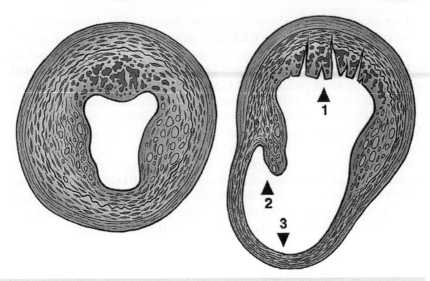

Fig. 2. Before (*left*) and after PTCA. Note the plaque rupture (*1*) and separation from intima (*2*), and stretching of less diseased artery (*3*). (*From* Landau C, Lange RA, Hillis LD. Percutaneous transluminal coronary angioplasty. N Engl J Med 1994;330:981, with permission. Copyright © 1994, Massachusetts Medical Society.)

of PCI compared with medical therapy and surgical management were cast in the spotlight.

Multiple therapies have been introduced as adjuncts to PCI in an attempt to decrease the rates of abrupt closure and restenosis. In the early 1980s Simpson

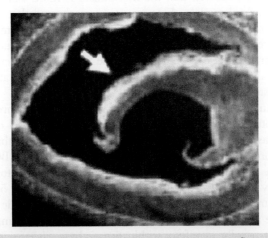

Fig. 3. Acute dissection after PTCA (*arrow*) denotes large coronary flap. (*From* Grech ED. Percutaneous coronary intervention. I: History and development. BMJ 2003;326:1080; with permission.)

modified an existing biopsy needle to create the first directional atherectomy catheter, with an aim of removing the existing plaque rather than dilating the vessel [13]. Along with rotational atherectomy and excimer laser ablation, directional atherectomy produced similar clinical results to PTCA and was more expensive, difficult to master, and had its own acute complications. In addition, the rate of restenosis was unchanged, requiring further TVR in the future [14]. A second approach to prevention of these complications was the placement of intravascular stents. Dotter and others had been experimenting with peripheral vascular stents since the late 1960s, and had explored materials such as stainless steel, nitinol (shape memory alloy), and even some silicone and plastics [1]. It was not until 1987, using a stainless steel, self-expanding device invented by Sigwart, that he and colleagues attempted the first human coronary stent placement (Fig. 4) [15].

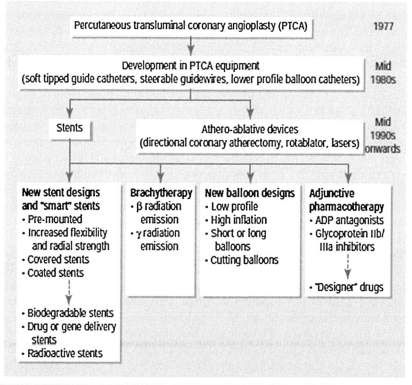

Fig. 4. Timeline of major events in PCI. (*From* National Institute of Neurologic Disorders, Stroke BM, Walker MD, et al. Executive Committee for the Asymptomatic Carotid Atherosclerosis Study: endarterectomy for asymptomatic carotid artery stenosis. JAMA 1995;273; with permission.)

BARE METAL STENTS

Sigwart and Puel developed their device with the intent of reducing restenosis as well as offering a percutaneous treatment of acute vessel dissection, which traditionally required emergency bypass surgery [3]. In the United States, the first devices approved by the Food and Drug Administration (FDA) were indicated for abrupt closure after PTCA [1]. Despite the limited indication, the placement of stents during PCI enjoyed a meteoric increase in the late 1980s to 1990s. As the first case series were released, it became apparent that these new devices, although they revolutionized the field, were fraught with their own complications. Early in-stent thrombosis (IST), caused by platelet adhesion to exposed metal struts (as well as acute plaque rupture from balloon angioplasty), complicated 10% to 20% of cases [16]. In addition, late restenosis, as neointimal proliferation obliterated the vessel lumen, continued to be a problem.

Bare metal stents (BMSs) clearly improved procedural success, and surgical standby, by offering interventionists a technique for opening vessels that had acutely occluded via dissection or acute thrombus formation. In addition, the luminal diameter was greater after stenting, likely because of a decrease in vessel wall elastic recoil [11]. Trials comparing PTCA and stenting, such as the STRESS (Stent Restenosis Study) and Benestent (Belgian Netherlands Stent Study) trials, showed that stents improved angiographic success and had a decrease in a composite end point of death, MI, and TVR (almost completely because of the decreased need for reintervention) [17,18]. This 10% decrease in the incidence of TVR was still present after 5 years [19]. These early trials had noted the risk of IST, which carries a mortality approaching 20% to 40% and MI rate of 45% [20]. Investigators adopted an intense anticoagulation regimen that often included preprocedural oral aspirin and dipyridamole, intravenous dextran and heparin, and continued oral warfarin therapy. This regimen was effective in reducing IST from 20% to between 3.5% and 10% but also resulted in an increase (from 3% to 13%) in bleeding complications, often involving the arterial access site [18]. Vascular surgery intervention was often necessary for pseudoaneurysm, arteriovenous fistula, and retroperitoneal hemorrhage.

The emergence of the thienopyridine class of antiplatelet medicines represents another step toward perfecting PCI. Thienopyridines, such as ticlopidine, inhibit adenosine diphosphate-mediated activation of the glycoprotein IIb/IIIa receptor, reducing platelet adhesion and aggregation [21]. Using dual antiplatelet therapy (DAPT) with aspirin and ticlopidine, researchers in the stent anticoagulation restinosis study (STARS) trial were able to show a reduction in IST to 0.5%, from close to 3% using aspirin and warfarin (Fig. 5). Hemorrhagic and vascular surgery complications occurred in 5.5% and 2% of cases, respectively, similar to the warfarin group [22]. Widespread use of ticlopidine revealed rare side effects of neutropenia and thrombotic thrombocytopenic pupura. This finding resulted in most practitioners switching to clopidogrel, another thienopyridine with a safer profile, and aspirin for DAPT. The most common DAPT regimen is aspirin plus clopidogrel, with a loading dose before the procedure, continued for 15 to 30 days after BMS [23]. Within 2 to 4 weeks

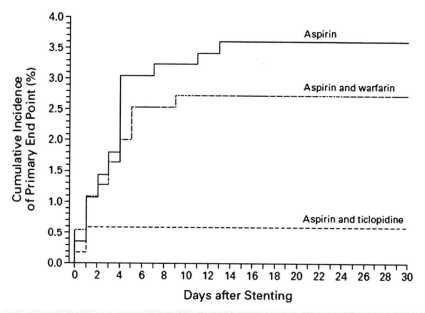

Fig. 5. Incidence of the primary end point in the 3 treatment groups in the STARS study. The primary end point was a composite of death, nonfatal MI, TVR, and IST on repeat angiogram. (*From* Leon MB, Baim DS, Popma JJ, et al. A clinical trial comparing three antithromboticdrug regimens after coronary-artery stenting. N Engl J Med 1998;339:1665; with permission. Copyright © 1998, Massachusetts Medical Society.)

of BMS placement, the metal struts become endothelialized and thrombogenic potential is vastly lower. Aspirin is typically recommended for life.

Using the new DAPT regimen, and taking advantage of other improvements in PCI technology such as stronger balloon materials (allowing higher inflation pressures), low-profile balloons and premounted, flexible stents (which allowed direct stenting rather than predilation followed by stent deployment), investigators looked again at the benefit of BMS over PTCA. The Benestent-II trial showed a decrease in major adverse cardiac events (MACEs) and higher 12-month incident-free survival in the BMS group [24]. This finding was largely a result of a reduced need for repeat PCI in the BMS group. As seen with previous studies, the initial cost and hospital length of stay were increased significantly after stent placement. The significance of the cost increase over time, because patients require repeated interventions after PTCA, is questionable.

The improved safety and usefulness of stents also allowed the comparison of PCI with the gold standard for cardiac revascularization, CABG. For patients with single-vessel disease, there may be a small survival advantage after PCI. However, there is an increased need for reintervention compared with CABG (Fig. 6) [25]. In the Stent or Surgery (SoS) trial, researchers compared BMS placement with CABG for multivessel disease. The incidence of death or MI was similar between groups, and the number of repeat revascularizations as a result

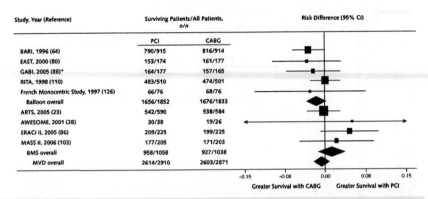

Fig. 6. Meta-analysis of trials comparing PCI (PTCA and BMS) with CABG. Five-year survival is equivalent between groups. Five-year survival with balloon angioplasty or stents versus CABG in patients with multivessel disease (MVD). The size of each box is proportional to the sample size of the trial. (*From* Perera GB, Lyden SP. Current trends in lower extremity revascularization. Surg Clin North Am 2007;87:1135; with permission.)

of late restenosis was significantly higher in the BMS group (21% vs 6% in the CABG group) [26]. There were significantly more deaths in the PCI group, a finding that was almost exclusively a result of cancer-related death [27].

Despite the advances in the technology of catheters, balloons, and stents, and improvements in periprocedural pharmacotherapy, PCI continued to be plagued by in-stent restenosis (ISR). Between 15% and 24% of patients develop late ISR after BMS; there is an even higher incidence in patients with diabetes [28]. Diffuse lesions can be particularly difficult to treat, which led many practitioners to call for provisional stenting (only for suboptimal results after PTCA) rather than primary stenting [29]. The cost-effectiveness of PCI with BMS over that of CABG was also called into question, because multiple stents were placed, and replaced, over the years. The culprit behind ISR, neointimal hyperproliferation, became the key target for improving outcomes. Multiple therapies including intravascular ultrasound guidance of stent placement, vascular brachytherapy (in-stent radiation), oral antiinflammatory drugs, covered stents, and drug-coated and drug-impregnated stents were explored. Of these therapies, drug-eluting stents (DESs) became the most widely used.

DESs

The concept behind DESs is that medicines that limit thrombosis and inflammation can be delivered directly to the site of vessel injury, at the time of the insult, and thereby reduce the initial hyperplastic response with minimal systemic drug exposure. The first devices were coated with heparin or dexamethasone, which had been shown to inhibit smooth muscle growth in vitro. However, the clinical success was disappointing, and they failed to significantly reduce neointimal proliferation [30]. The next round of drugs showed more promise. Laboratory studies showed that hydrophilic drugs, such as heparin, failed to adequately penetrate the tissue surrounding the stent [30]. In addition, they were not present in therapeutic concentrations long enough to make a significant impact. Paclitaxel and sirolimus, drugs that had been used for chemotherapy and immunosuppression, respectively, came to the forefront. These drugs are hydrophobic, allowing them to penetrate tissue more easily, and they are imbedded in a polymer coating that allows for controlled release.

The sirolimus-eluting stents were the first to be widely tested, and initial results were promising. Results from the randomized study with the sirolimus-coated Bx velocity balloon-expandable stent in the treatment of patients with de novo native coronary artery lesions trial showed a significant reduction in MACE, fueled entirely by the decreased incidence in TVR (22% after BMS, and none in the DES group) [31]. Other studies echoed these findings, and the overall incidence of TVR was around 5% after DES and 15% after BMS [32]. This finding is compared with the 30% TVR rate after PTCA. These findings were enthusiastically embraced by the interventional community, despite the lack of long-term outcomes data, and the use of DES became rampant. Although the FDA indication is for short de novo lesions in patients with symptomatic ischemia, clinicians used them in a variety of off-label situations. They proved to be effective in patients with acute MI [33], to treat multivessel and diffuse lesions, to treat ISR with BMS [34], and to treat saphenous vein grafts stenosis. From 2003 to 2004, use skyrocketed from 19.7% to 78.2% of percutaneous coronary procedures [35].

Clinicians recognized the threat of subacute IST, because the antiproliferative drugs prevented new intimal growth, resulting in a longer exposure period of the metal struts to the circulation. Therefore most patients were kept on DAPT for 2 to 6 months (instead of the 15–30 days for BMS). After this period, it was hoped that the polymer coating on the stents would be deplete of agent, and normal endothelialization would occur. The sirolimus stent was predicted to elute 80% of its drug by 30 days, and the paclitaxel stent by 90 days [36]. However, as long-term data were published, clinicians discovered that the window for IST, which carries a significant risk for death or MI, extended later than anticipated. Reports of late IST began to emerge, causing the FDA to issue warnings, and creating panic among clinicians and patients. The perception was of a ticking time bomb in the chest of patients with DES. Autopsy reports supported these findings [36], and reported significantly delayed arterial wall healing with DES compared with BMS. In addition, many of these cases seemed to be temporally related to cessation of DAPT, which led clinicians to extend the regimen to 12 months [23]. Some even recommended lifetime DAPT, because the optimal treatment course was unknown.

Longer-term (4 and 5 years) data from randomized controlled trials and registries are now available, and the results seem to mitigate some of the fear surrounding DES. The annual incidence of IST for DES seems to be around 0.6% to 1% [37], similar to rates of IST after BMS placement [38]. These studies reinforce that IST is associated with high morbidity and mortality. They also support DAPT for at least 12 months, because many cases of IST were noted to have stopped therapy [39,40]. However, after 1 year, doubt still lingers as to whether DAPT or monotherapy is more appropriate. Histologic data have shown that, beyond 30 days, DESs, ironically, provoke a greater inflammatory response than BMS with more eosinophils, giant cells, and fibrin deposition around struts, leading to poor vessel healing [36]. This finding may be a response to the polymer coating rather than the drug, which has a limited period of activity [41]. Another confounder of the IST issue is the newly realized problem of clopidogrel resistance, which may have an incidence of close to 20% and increase the risk for IST (Figs. 7 and 8) [42].

FUTURE DIRECTIONS

Soon, we will begin seeing the results of trials using a second generation of DES. These trials will use newer alloys, new analogues of sirolimus and paclitaxel, and newer, biodegradable polymer coatings. Some will try to combine drugs, and some will avoid the polymer debate by embedding drug directly into the metal frame of the stent. These stents will all still suffer from the problem of foreign metal interacting with tissue, resulting in abnormal wound healing [43]. As with BMS, when antiplatelet therapy is withdrawn, the patient is at risk for thrombotic events [44]. A different approach is the biodegradable polymer-based stent. The theory is that a fully absorbable, DES limits

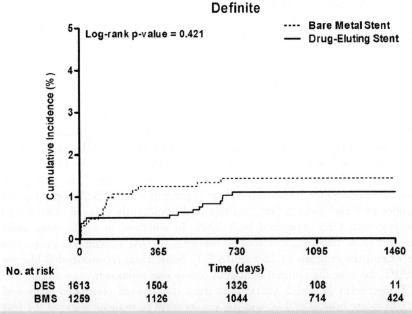

Fig. 7. Kaplan-Meier curve depicting cumulative incidence of definite IST, as defined by the Academic Research Consortium, with DES and BMS. (*From* Applegate RJ, Sacrinty MT, Little WC, et al. Incidence of coronary stent thrombosis based on academic research consortium definitions. Am J Cardiol 2008;102:683; with permission.)

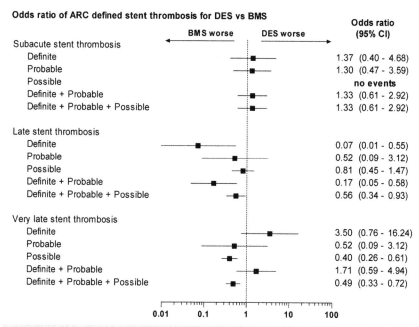

Fig. 8. OR plot of Academic Research Consortium-defined IST for DES-treated and BMS-treated patients in 3 different time intervals. (*From* Applegate RJ, Sacrinty MT, Little WC, et al. Incidence of coronary stent thrombosis based on academic research consortium definitions. Am J Cardiol 2008;102:683; with permission.)

neointimal proliferation and elastic recoil during the acute phase, and is eventually absorbed into the vessel wall, limiting the long-term thrombogenic potential. A small trial of an everolimus-eluting bioabsorbable stent reported success [45], but larger randomized controlled trials are needed.

In the meantime, PCI must focus on tailoring interventions to each individual patient. Platelet aggregation assays can predict clopidogrel-resistant patients, who may benefit from other thienopyridines such as prasugrel. Not only is prasugrel effective for patients with a poor response to clopidogrel but it may be more effective in patients with diabetes and those presenting with STEMI (ST elevation MI) [46]. In addition, the optimal treatment duration of antiplatelet therapy is yet to be determined. Practitioners must also determine when and where to use these different therapies. Challenging clinical scenarios such as bifurcation lesions [47], saphenous vein graft stenosis [48], patients on oral anticoagulant therapy (such as with warfarin), and diffuse multivessel disease still await the definitive answer.

PERIOPERATIVE MANAGEMENT OF ANGIOPLASTY PATIENTS

Before the advent of coronary stents in the early 1990s, PTCA was the mainstay of nonsurgical revascularization despite a 30% to 50% incidence of restenosis, most often occurring within 3 months [49] and frequently requiring repeat procedures [50]. After balloon angioplasty, patients typically maintained antiplatelet therapy with aspirin for 4 to 6 weeks to prevent rethrombosis. Multiple, small retrospective analyses of patients receiving angioplasty before noncardiac surgery failed to identify a significantly increased risk of death or cardiac event [51–53]. However, a larger, retrospective study reported an increased risk of mortality and perioperative MI in patients receiving angioplasty within 2 weeks before surgery. An analysis of the Mayo Clinic Percutaneous Coronary Intervention and General Surgery databases identified 345 patients undergoing 350 angioplasty procedures within 60 days before surgery [54]. All 3 patients who suffered death or MI had their angioplasty performed less than 2 weeks before surgery. An additional 9 episodes of repeat revascularization were necessary in patients who had angioplasty 3 to 7 weeks before surgery. No incidents of death, MI, or repeat revascularization occurred in patients receiving angioplasty greater than 7 weeks before surgery. However, there is a theoretic concern that delaying elective surgery greater than 8 weeks after balloon angioplasty may be associated with increased risk of perioperative ischemia caused by possible restenosis. Therefore the American College of Cardiology (ACC) and American Heart Association (AHA) 2009 *Guidelines on Perioperative Cardiovascular Evaluation and Care for Noncardiac Surgery* recommends 4 to 6 weeks of antiplatelet therapy with aspirin and delaying surgery at least 2 weeks but not greater than 8 weeks after balloon angioplasty (Fig. 9) [23].

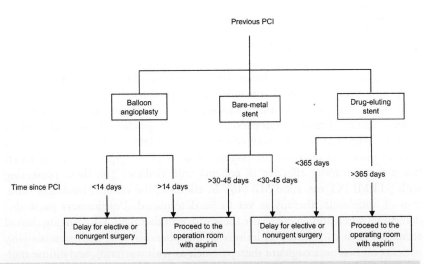

Fig. 9. Proposed approach to the management of patients with previous PCI requiring noncardiac surgery (based on expert opinion). (*From* Fleisher LA, Beckman JA, Brown KA, et al. 2009 ACCF/AHA focused update on perioperative beta blockade incorporated into the ACC/AHA 2007 guidelines on perioperative cardiovascular evaluation and care for noncardiac surgery: a report of the American College of Cardiology Foundation/American Heart Association Task Force on practice guidelines. Circulation 2009;120:e169; with permission.)

PERIOPERATIVE MANAGEMENT OF PATIENTS WITH BMSS

Because of the high rate of early reocclusion and late restenosis, the use of balloon angioplasty has declined, and coronary artery stents were developed to maintain better vessel patency. However, the prothrombotic milieu of the perioperative experience, stemming from withholding of anticoagulation and antiplatelet medication preoperatively, surgical-induced release of proinflammatory and prothrombotic mediators, and frequent postoperative immobility, increases the possibility of thrombotic events. Retrospective data collected at the Mayo Clinic identified a significantly increased incidence of MACEs (death, MI, stent thrombosis, or repeat revascularization with either CABG or PCI of the target vessel) in patients who underwent noncardiac surgery less than 30 days after PCI with BMS (Figs. 10 and 11) [55–58]. Because of the increased incidence of perioperative complications, the ACC/AHA recommend DAPT with aspirin and clopidogrel for 4 to 6 weeks and delaying elective surgery after BMS (See Fig. 9). Much of the controversy regarding perioperative management of patients with BMSs surrounds the management

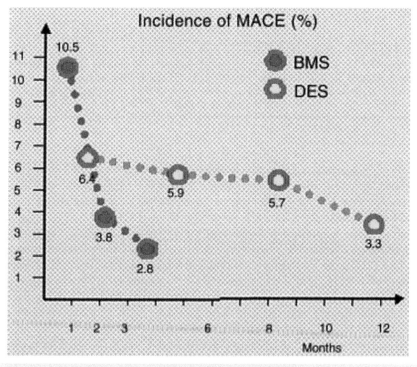

Fig. 10. Incidence of MACEs according to delay (months) between stent implantation and noncardiac surgery. Events include MI, stent thrombosis, TVI, and death. (*From* Eberli D, Chassot PG, Sulser T, et al. Urological surgery and antiplatelet drugs after cardiac and cerebrovascular accidents. J Urol 2010;183:2128; with permission.)

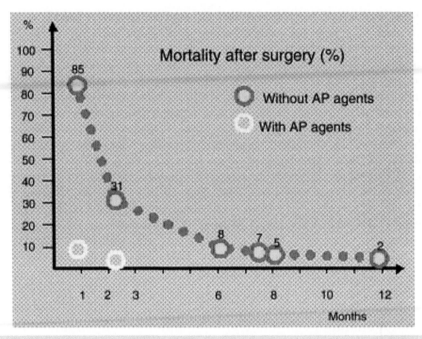

Fig. 11. Mortality of patients with coronary stents taken off antiplatelet drugs for noncardiac surgery according to delay since coronary revascularization. Two studies have comparative data on mortality of patients operated on without cessation of antiplatelet drugs (5% and 0%, respectively). (*From* Eberli D, Chassot PG, Sulser T, et al. Urological surgery and antiplatelet drugs after cardiac and cerebrovascular accidents. J Urol 2010;183:2128; with permission.)

of newly diagnosed significant coronary artery disease (CAD) during the preoperative evaluation of patients for noncardiac surgery. Should these patients receive coronary stents preoperatively to reduce the incidence of perioperative MI? Can the noncardiac surgery be delayed at least 4 to 6 weeks after stenting to allow appropriate antiplatelet therapy to reduce IST?

PCI for coronary revascularization before noncardiac surgery has decreased in light of 2 large multicenter, randomized trials reporting no benefit when compared with medical management [59,60]. With nearly a 50% incidence of CAD, high-risk vascular surgery patients have been studied for risk modification before elective surgery [61]. The Coronary Artery Revascularization Prophylaxis (CARP) and Dutch Echocardiographic Cardiac Risk Evaluation Applying Stress Echo Study Group (DECREASE-V) trials compared coronary revascularization with medical management in patients scheduled for elective abdominal aortic or aortoiliac surgery. The CARP trial compared both PCI with DES or CABG with medical management and reported no difference in the primary outcome of mortality after nearly 3 years of follow-up. The mortality was 22% in the revascularization group, versus 23% with medical management (relative risk, 0.98; 95% confidence interval [CI], 0.70–1.37; $P = .92$). In addition, the incidence of postoperative MI was similar between the 2 groups (12% vs 14%, $P = .37$). However there was a difference between the number of vessels revascularized with PCI and CABG (1.3 ± 0.8 vs 3.0 ± 0.8) and the timing of revascularization (1 vs 18 days) (Fig. 12).

The DECREASE-V trial pilot study compared PCI or CABG with medical management in patients scheduled for elective major vascular surgery and reported similar results to the CARP trial. There was no difference between revascularization and medical management in 30-day (HR, 2.2; 95% CI, 0.74–6.6; $P = .14$) and 1-year all-cause mortality (hazard ratio [HR], 1.3; 95% CI, 0.55–2.9; $P = .58$). In addition, there was no difference in the composite outcome of mortality and nonfatal MI at 30 days and 1 year after vascular surgery. In a subsequent publication, the Dutch group found no benefit to revascularization after long-term follow-up (median follow-up 2.8 years) after vascular surgery [62].

Evaluation of the effect of PCI on postoperative outcomes is difficult because both the CARP and DECREASE-V trials included patients randomized to surgical revascularization via CABG. However, in a meta-analysis of the trials, Biccard and Rodseth evaluated the primary outcomes of mortality and postoperative MI according to type of coronary revascularization performed [63]. In

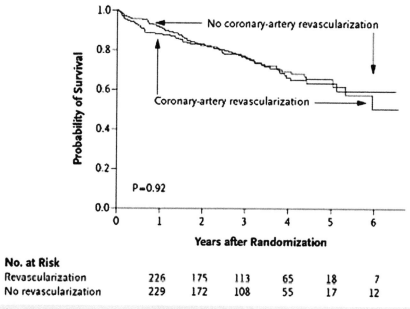

No. at Risk

Revascularization	226	175	113	65	18	7
No revascularization	229	172	108	55	17	12

Fig. 12. Long-term survival among patients assigned to undergo coronary-artery revascularization or no coronary-artery revascularization before elective major vascular surgery. (*From* McFalls EO, Ward HB, Moritz TE, et al. Coronary-artery revascularization before elective major vascular surgery. N Engl J Med 2004;351:2795; with permission. Copyright © 2009, Massachusetts Medical Society.)

these investigators' analysis, patients who received PCI compared with medical management developed a nonsignificant trend toward increased 30-day all-cause mortality (odds ratio [OR], 1.68; 95% CI, 0.78–3.62; $P = .18$) and significant trend toward increased 30-day nonfatal MI (OR 2.14; 95% CI, 1.05–4.36; $P = .04$). In light of the CARP and DECREASE-V trials, the usefulness of preoperative revascularization before major surgery is questionable for both short-term and long-term outcomes (Fig. 13).

PERIOPERATIVE MANAGEMENT OF PATIENTS WITH DESs

Because of the increased risk of late IST, patients receiving DESs are required to remain compliant with aspirin and clopidogrel DAPT for at least 12 months and typically longer. In addition to a reduced rate of revascularization, the Clopidogrel for the Reduction of Events During Observation (CREDO) trial demonstrated that 12 months of clopidogrel, versus aspirin alone, lead to a reduction in the one-year composite end point of death, MI and stroke [64]. Therefore, the ACC/AHA recommend DAPT with aspirin and clopidogrel for at least 12 months after DES to reduce the risk of IST (see Fig. 9). Based on the increased bleeding risk associated with clopidogrel in multiple studies, cessation of clopidogrel is advised to reduce perioperative bleeding, improve surgical hemostasis, and reduce transfusion requirements. A meta analysis of 18 large trials comprising nearly 130,000 patients documented a 47% increased incidence of major bleeding, although no difference was seen in fatal or intracranial bleeds [65]. In a cardiac surgery meta-analysis, there are fairly consistent data showing increased chest tube output, increased reexploration rate, and

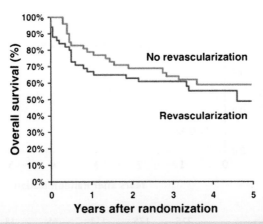

Fig. 13. Overall survival in 101 randomly assigned patients to no preoperative coronary revascularization versus patients assigned to preoperative coronary revascularization before major vascular surgery. (*From* Schouten O, van Kuijk JP, Flu WJ, et al. Long-term outcome of prophylactic coronary revascularization in cardiac high-risk patients undergoing major vascular surgery (from the Randomized DECREASE-V Pilot Study). Am J Cardiol 2009;103:897; with permission.)

increased transfusion requirements in patients receiving clopidogrel less than 5 days before CABG. However, there was no significant increase in hospital length of stay or mortality [66]. In noncardiac surgery, in which the likelihood of bleeding is less, the risk of increased perioperative bleeding because of DAPT is less clear. A review of more than 10,000 patients in the New England Vascular Surgery Database did not show increased postoperative bleeding associated with specific antiplatelet therapy [67]. The investigators' review of prospectively obtained data reported no difference in the rate of reoperation for bleeding (1.5%, 1.3%, 0.9%, 1.5%; $P = .74$); incidence of transfusion (18%, 17%, 0%, 24%; $P = .1$); and transfusion requirements (0.7 units, 0.5 units, 0 units, 0.6 units; $P = .1$).

Although there is controversy regarding the degree of increased perioperative bleeding associated with DAPT, that associated with aspirin therapy alone is likely significantly less. A small study of 52 patients undergoing emergency surgery did not reveal an increase in perioperative bleeding [68]. However, a later meta-analysis showed an increased rate of perioperative bleeding complications by a factor of 1.5; the level of severity of bleeding complications was not greater (except for intracranial surgery and prostatectomy) [69]. There is no evidence showing aspirin use increases the risk of epidural hematoma from neuraxial anesthesia [70]. Aspirin therapy should be stopped only if the risk of perioperative bleeding exceeds the risk of cardiac complications caused by aspirin withdrawal.

An approach to balance the risk of perioperative bleeding associated with DAPT in patients with a recent DES versus the risk of IST is to stop clopidogrel 5 to 7 days preoperatively, and treat the patient with intravenous IIb/IIIa inhibitor until the time of surgery. There are few data showing the benefits of antiplatelet bridging therapy in noncardiac surgery. A phase II trial of tirofiban bridging therapy in 30 patients with recent DES reported no cases of death, MI, revascularization, or reexploration for surgical bleeding [71]. The investigators report 1 episode of major and minor bleeding and 4 patients receiving transfusion. Antiplatelet bridging therapy started 24 hours after withdrawal of clopidogrel until the time of surgery, and may improve surgical bleeding risk without significantly increasing thrombotic complications. In addition, resuming antiplatelet therapy as soon as possible postoperatively with either IIb/IIIa inhibitors or clopidogrel loading has been recommended.

Delaying urgent surgery for patients on DAPT for a recent DES to allow improvement in platelet function is controversial because of the competing risks of IST and bleeding, which must be balanced against the possible consequences associated with delay of surgery and worsening of the surgical disease. Frequently this dilemma occurs in patients treated with clopidogrel who fall and suffer a hip fracture requiring urgent intervention. Delaying repair of hip fracture greater than 48 hours may increase the risks of perioperative complications and mortality. Recent investigations have evaluated the incidence of perioperative bleeding in patients maintained on clopidogrel versus those not [72]. In a prospective, case-control trial of 88 patients, the investigators reported total blood loss was significantly greater in patients treated with clopidogrel, with or without aspirin, versus those not taking clopidogrel (1312 ± 686 mL, 1091 ± 654 mL, 899 ± 496 mL, respectively). The increased incidence of major complications (5 episodes of acute coronary syndrome, 2 cardiovascular accidents), 6 of which occurred in patients maintained on clopidogrel, was likely caused by the higher prevalence of comorbidities among patients treated with clopidogrel.

Patients with recent DES and receiving DAPT may present for lower extremity revascularization or urological surgery amenable to neuraxial anesthesia. Despite specific evidence showing increased risk of spinal hematoma, the recent American Society of Regional Anesthesia (ASRA) 2010 Guidelines continue to recommend withholding thienopyridines, such as clopidogrel and ticlopidine, 7 days before neuraxial anesthesia [73]. If a patient has been treated with a IIb/IIIa inhibitor as bridging therapy, discontinuation is advised 24 to 48 hours before surgery for abciximab and 4 to 8 hours for eptifibatide and tirofiban, with frequent neurologic assessments postoperatively. Aspirin cessation is not recommended before neuraxial anesthesia. Although no data exist, the ASRA guidelines suggest similar management for patients receiving deep plexus or peripheral nerve blockade.

The management of patients with severe perioperative bleeding in the setting of DAPT for recent DES implantation has not been well studied. Because of the irreversible nature of platelet inhibition by aspirin and thienopyridines, a significant number of platelet transfusions may be necessary to reduce serious complications such as intracranial bleeding. Adjunctive therapy may include desmopressin, antifibrinolytics, and recombinant factor VIIa [74].

ANTIPLATELET AGENT PHARMACOLOGY

Recent reviews have provided extensive updates of the pharmacology of antiplatelet agents, which are the mainstay of preventing coronary artery thrombosis and coronary stent restenosis (Fig. 14 and Table 1) [75,76]. Three classes of antiplatelet agents are commonly used clinically: aspirin, thienopyridines, and glycoprotein IIb/IIIa inhibitors. Aspirin, the most common antiplatelet agent used, irreversibly inhibits cyclooxygenase 1 (COX-1) by acetylation, thereby decreasing thromboxane A_2 (TXA_2) synthesis and consequently TXA_2-induced platelet activation and aggregation. The clinical half-life of aspirin is 5 to 6 days because of the time necessary for generation of new platelets.

The second class of antiplatelet agents, often used in combination with aspirin, are thienopyridines: ticlopidine and clopidogrel, and recently prasugrel and ticagrelor. These agents inhibit $P2Y_{12}$, and thus adenosine diphosphate (ADP) receptor-mediated platelet activation. Ticlopidine is rarely used clinically because of inconvenient twice-daily dosing and a serious side effect profile, including thrombocytopenia purpura and bone marrow aplasia. Clopidogrel, the most commonly used $P2Y_{12}$ inhibitor, irreversibly blocks ADP-mediated platelet activation, but is limited by unpredictable conversion from prodrug form to active metabolite via a 2-step process, resulting in variable

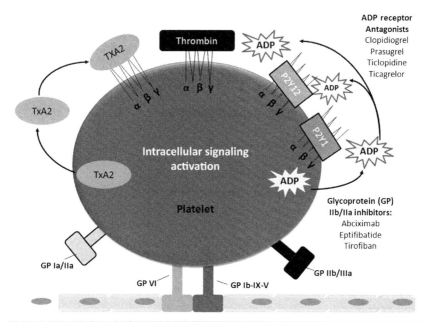

Fig. 14. Targets for antiplatelet therapy. (*From* Uren N. Acute coronary syndromes: assessing risk and choosing optimal pharmacologic regimens for a superior outcome. Eur Heart J Suppl 2010;12:D4; with permission.)

clinical response and many nonresponders [77]. The more recently developed prasugrel requires only 1 step conversion to active metabolite and is associated with more rapid onset and greater clinical efficacy in phase II clinical trials [78]. Because of the greater degree of platelet inhibition by prasugrel versus clopidogrel, patients presenting for surgery may require withholding prasugrel for a greater period of time, when clinically indicated. An investigational $P2Y_{12}$ antagonist, ticagrelor, may offer advantages over the previous agents because of its direct action and reversible inhibition of the $P2Y_{12}$ receptor.

Table 1			
Summary of antiplatelet agents			
	Mechanism of action	Biologic half-life	Common adverse reactions
Aspirin	COX-1 inhibition	Life of platelets (7–10 d)	Gastrointestinal intolerance, bleeding, allergy
Clopidogrel	ADP receptor inhibition	5–6 d	P450 drug metabolism
Prasugrel	ADP receptor inhibition	5–10 d	Bleeding in age ≥75 y and body weight <60 kg
Abciximab	Glycoprotein IIb/IIIa inhibition	24–48 h	Bleeding, thrombocytopenia
Tirofiban	Glycoprotein IIb/IIIa inhibition	4–8 h	Bleeding
Eptifibatide	Glycoprotein IIb/IIIa inhibition	4–8 h	Bleeding

The last class of commonly used antiplatelet agents are glycoprotein IIb/IIIa inhibitors used during PCI to potently block platelet activity, but carry a greater risk of bleeding and thrombocytopenia. Tirofiban and eptifibatide have a shorter half-life than the abciximab, a Fab fragment specific for the IIb/IIIa receptor, but are renally cleared and may require dose adjustment in kidney disease [79–81].

CAROTID ANGIOPLASTY AND STENTING

In the United States there are about 600,000 new strokes per year (about 1 every 52 seconds). Stroke is the third leading cause of death and a leading cause of long-term disability in the United States, with direct and indirect costs of about $74 billion per year [82]. Three large prospective randomized trials have clearly shown that carotid endarterectomy (CEA) is the gold standard for symptomatic and asymptomatic patients with carotid artery stenosis. The European Carotid Surgery Trial (ECST) showed that in patients with transient ischemic accident or stroke and ipsilateral carotid artery stenosis greater than 80%, CEA decreased the risk of ipsilateral stroke from 20.6% to 6.8% ($P<.0001$) when compared with best medical treatment (BMT) [83]. Similar results were found in the North American Symptomatic Carotid Endarterectomy Trial [84,85]. In this trial symptomatic patients with severe carotid artery stenosis (70%–99%) treated with CEA had a risk of stroke of 9% at 2 years versus 26% in the BMT ($P<.001$) [84]. Furthermore, patients with 50% to 69% stenosis also benefited from CEA, with a 5-year stroke risk of 15.7% in the CEA group versus 22.2% in the BMT group ($P = .045$) [85].

Three large prospective trials have evaluated the role of CEA in patients with asymptomatic carotid artery disease. The Veterans Affairs Cooperative Trial (VACT) showed that in asymptomatic male patients with carotid stenosis greater than 50% the risk of stroke was 8.0% versus 20.6% at 47.9 months ($P \leq .001$) in the CEA versus BMT groups [86]. The Asymptomatic Carotid Atherosclerosis Study (ACAS) showed similar results with a reduction in 5-year stroke or death rate of 5.1% in the CEA group versus 11% in the BMT group ($P = .004$) [87]. The Asymptomatic Carotid Surgery Trial (ACST) showed a decreased 5-year stroke rate of 6.4% versus 11.8% in the BMT group ($P<.0001$) [88].

Based on these trials the AHA treatment guidelines recommend CEA in symptomatic patients with greater than 50% stenosis if the perioperative risk of stroke or death is less than 6% [89]. It is important to recognize that all 6 of these trials enrolled a limited subset of mostly low-risk surgical patients, and the procedures were performed by skilled surgeons at highly selected institutions. For example, 25 patients were screened for each 1 patient enrolled in the ACAS trial [82,90]. In addition, there have been tremendous advancements in the BMT since these trials were conducted in the 1980s and 1990s [91–94].

To further muddy the waters, several studies of carotid artery stenting (CAS) have been reported. The first carotid artery balloon angioplasty was performed in 1979 [95], and since then there have been many single-center and multicenter prospective randomized trials of CEA versus CAS. The results of these trials have been reviewed in 2 articles [82,96]. Recently, the results of 2 large prospective studies comparing CEA with CAS have been published. The International Carotid Stenting Study (ICSS) evaluated patients with symptomatic carotid artery disease and carotid stenosis greater than 50% who were randomized to CEA or CAS. Stroke, death, or MI at 120 days was 8.5% in the CAS group versus 5.2% in the CEA group ($P = .0006$) [97]. The Carotid Revascularization Endarterectomy versus Stenting Trial (CREST), which included both symptomatic and asymptomatic patients with carotid artery stenosis, showed that at 2.5 years the incidence of death, stroke, or MI was not different between groups (7.2% vs 6.8%, CAS vs CEA, $P = .51$) [98]. The 4-year rate of stroke or death was 6.4% with CAS versus 4.7% with CEA ($P = .03$).

A systematic review and meta-analysis of CEA versus CAS using 11 trials of 4796 patients showed that the 30-day risk of death or stroke was lower in the CEA group (95% CI, 0.47–0.95, $P = .025$), (Fig. 15); however, there was no difference in death or stroke at 1 to 4 years (95% CI, 0.74–1.1%, $P = .314$) (Fig. 16) [99].

Antiplatelet therapy has also evolved over time. The recently reported CREST Trial required that all patients undergoing CAS receive DAPT before the procedure and at least 30 days after the procedure [97]. Most patients stay

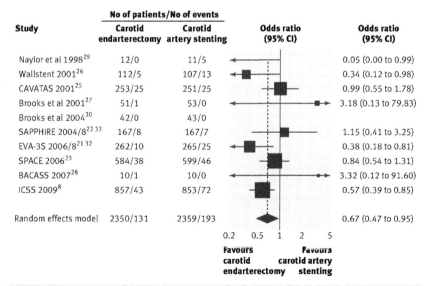

Fig. 15. Forest plot of ORs of risk for composite of stroke or death within 30 days of CEA versus CAS. (*From* Meier P, Knapp G, Tamhane U, et al. Short term and intermediate term comparison of endarterectomy versus stenting for carotid artery stenosis: systematic review and metaanalysis of randomised controlled clinical trials. BMJ 2010;340:c467; with permission.)

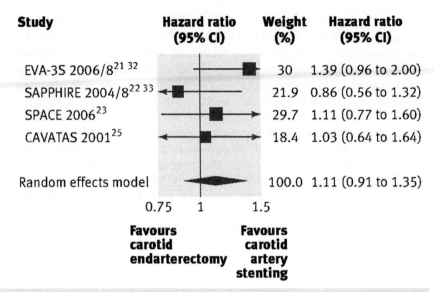

Fig. 16. Forest plot of HR of intermediate-term risk for composite of stroke or death. (*From* Meier P, Knapp G, Tamhane U, et al. Short term and intermediate term comparison of endarterectomy versus stenting for carotid artery stenosis: systematic review and metaanalysis of randomised controlled clinical trials. BMJ 2010;340:c467; with permission.)

on acetylsalicylic acid (ASA) or clopidogrel for life. There have been case reports of in-stent carotid occlusion after premature discontinuation of DAPT [100]. Because of this finding, it is prudent to follow similar recommendations for BMS in the coronary arteries: delay elective surgery for 30 to 45 days of DAPT after CAS, then perform the procedure while on DAPT or ASA alone if risk of procedural bleeding is low. If ASA is stopped it should be restarted as soon as possible. For procedures that cannot be delayed 30 to 45 days, the risk of stroke versus the risk of procedural bleeding must be individualized, and the use of short-acting antiplatelet therapy (llb/llla inhibitors) could be considered.

PERIPHERAL VASCULAR DISEASE AND STENTING

The use of endovascular stents continues to evolve in the management of peripheral and mesenteric artery disease [101–104]. However, there is considerable variability in the management of antiplatelet therapy in the perioperative period. The most conservative approach is to follow the guidelines for anticoagulation for BMS or DES in the coronary circulation. However, many radiologists and endovascular surgeons do not routinely use DAPT after peripheral aortic stenting. Because of the lack of data and consensus regarding peripheral vascular stents, we recommend perioperative discussion with the interventionists and the surgeon to individualize the perioperative antiplatelet regimen.

SUMMARY

Interventional cardiology, radiology, and endovascular surgery procedures continue to evolve and advance, with constant changes and improvements in technology. Antiplatelet pharmacology and best medical practices for patients with atherosclerotic vascular disease are also continuously changing. Because of this situation, perioperative patients should be optimized to best medical practice, and the risks of bleeding versus thrombosis must be weighed for each patient.

References

[1] Mueller RL, Sanborn TA. The history of interventional cardiology: cardiac catheterization, angioplasty, and related interventions. Am Heart J 1995;129:146.

[2] Gruentzig AR, Senning Āk, Siegenthaler WE. Nonoperative dilatation of coronary-artery stenosis. N Engl J Med 1979;301:61.

[3] Douglas JS, King SB. Hurst's the heart. 10th edition. New York (NY): McGraw-Hill; 2001. p. 1437.

[4] Hueb WA, Bellotti G, de Oliveira SA, et al. The Medicine, Angioplasty or Surgery Study (MASS): a prospective, randomized trial of medical therapy, balloon angioplasty or bypass surgery for single proximal left anterior descending artery stenoses. J Am Coll Cardiol 1995;26:1600.

[5] Coronary angioplasty versus medical therapy for angina: the second Randomised Intervention Treatment of Angina (RITA-2) trial. Lancet 1997;350:461.

[6] Hueb W, Soares PR, Gersh BJ, et al. The medicine, angioplasty, or surgery study (MASS-II): a randomized, controlled clinical trial of three therapeutic strategies for multivessel coronary artery disease: one-year results. J Am Coll Cardiol 2004;43:1743.

[7] Participants RT. Coronary angioplasty versus coronary artery bypass surgery: the Randomised Intervention Treatment of Angina (RITA) trial. Lancet 1993;341:573.

[8] King SB, Lembo NJ, Weintraub WS, et al. A randomized trial comparing coronary angioplasty with coronary bypass surgery. N Engl J Med 1994;331:1044.

[9] Mathew JP, Fontes ML, Tudor IC, et al. A multicenter risk index for atrial fibrillation after cardiac surgery. JAMA 2004;291:1720.

[10] Castaneda-Zuniga WR, Formanek A, Tadavarthy M, et al. The mechanism of balloon angioplasty. Radiology 1980;135:565.

[11] Grech ED. Percutaneous coronary intervention. I: History and development. BMJ 2003;326:1080.

[12] Morrison DA. Stent thrombosis: the effect of intention on perception. J Am Coll Cardiol 2010;55:1943.

[13] Simpson JB, Selmon MR, Robertson GC, et al. Transluminal atherectomy for occlusive peripheral vascular disease. Am J Cardiol 1988;61:96G.

[14] Adelman AG, Cohen EA, Kimball BP, et al. A comparison of directional atherectomy with balloon angioplasty for lesions of the left anterior descending coronary artery. N Engl J Med 1993;329:228.

[15] Sigwart U, Puel J, Mirkovitch V, et al. Intravascular stents to prevent occlusion and restenosis after transluminal angioplasty. N Engl J Med 1987;316:701.

[16] Serruys PW, Strauss BH, Beatt KJ, et al. Angiographic follow-up after placement of a self-expanding coronary-artery stent. N Engl J Med 1991;324:13.

[17] Fischman DL, Leon MB, Baim DS, et al. A randomized comparison of coronary-stent placement and balloon angioplasty in the treatment of coronary artery disease. N Engl J Med 1994;331:496.

[18] Serruys PW, de Jaegere P, Kiemeneij F, et al. A comparison of balloon-expandable-stent implantation with balloon angioplasty in patients with coronary artery disease. N Engl J Med 1994;331:489.

[19] Kiemeneij F, Serruys PW, Macaya C, et al. Continued benefit of coronary stenting versus balloon angioplasty: five-year clinical follow-up of Benestent-I trial. J Am Coll Cardiol 2001;37:1598.

[20] Urban P, Gershlick AH, Guagliumi G, et al. Safety of coronary sirolimus-eluting stents in daily clinical practice: one-year follow-up of the e-Cypher registry. Circulation 2006;113:1434.

[21] Calver AL, Blows LJ, Harmer S, et al. Clopidogrel for prevention of major cardiac events after coronary stent implantation: 30-day and 6-month results in patients with smaller stents. Am Heart J 2000;140:483.

[22] Leon MB, Baim DS, Popma JJ, et al. A clinical trial comparing three antithrombotic-drug regimens after coronary-artery stenting. N Engl J Med 1998;339:1665.

[23] Fleisher LA, Beckman JA, Brown KA, et al. ACC/AHA 2007 guidelines on perioperative cardiovascular evaluation and care for noncardiac surgery: executive summary: a report of the American College of Cardiology/American Heart Association Task Force on Practice Guidelines (Writing Committee to Revise the 2002 Guidelines on Perioperative Cardiovascular Evaluation for Noncardiac Surgery) Developed in Collaboration with the American Society of Echocardiography, American Society of Nuclear Cardiology, Heart Rhythm Society, Society of Cardiovascular Anesthesiologists, Society for Cardiovascular Angiography and Interventions, Society for Vascular Medicine and Biology, and Society for Vascular Surgery. J Am Coll Cardiol 2007;50:1707.

[24] Serruys PW, van Hout B, Bonnier H, et al. Randomised comparison of implantation of heparin-coated stents with balloon angioplasty in selected patients with coronary artery disease (Benestent II). Lancet 1998;352:673.

[25] Bravata DM, Gienger AL, McDonald KM, et al. Systematic review: the comparative effectiveness of percutaneous coronary interventions and coronary artery bypass graft surgery. Ann Intern Med 2007;147:703.

[26] SoS Investigators. Coronary artery bypass surgery versus percutaneous coronary intervention with stent implantation in patients with multivessel coronary artery disease (the Stent or Surgery trial): a randomised controlled trial. Lancet 2002;360:965.

[27] Booth J, Clayton T, Pepper J, et al. Randomized, controlled trial of coronary artery bypass surgery versus percutaneous coronary intervention in patients with multivessel coronary artery disease: six-year follow-up from the Stent or Surgery trial (SoS). Circulation 2008;118:381.

[28] Stenestrand U, James SK, Lindbäck J, et al. Safety and efficacy of drug-eluting vs. bare metal stents in patients with diabetes mellitus: long-term follow-up in the Swedish Coronary Angiography and Angioplasty Registry (SCAAR). Eur Heart J 2010;31:177.

[29] Rupprecht HJ, Meyer J. A plea for provisional stenting. Eur Heart J 1999;20:1769.

[30] Hwang CW, Wu D, Edelman ER. Physiological transport forces govern drug distribution for stent-based delivery. Circulation 2001;104:600.

[31] Morice MC, Serruys PW, Sousa JE, et al. A randomized comparison of a sirolimus-eluting stent with a standard stent for coronary revascularization. N Engl J Med 2002;346:1773.

[32] Roiron C, Sanchez P, Bouzamondo A, et al. Drug eluting stents: an updated meta-analysis of randomised controlled trials. Heart 2006;92:641.

[33] Kupferwasser LI, Amorn AM, Kapoor N, et al. Comparison of drug-eluting stents with bare metal stents in unselected patients with acute myocardial infarction. Catheter Cardiovasc Interv 2007;70:1.

[34] Holmes DR, Teirstein P, Satler L, et al. Sirolimus-eluting stents vs vascular brachytherapy for in-stent restenosis within bare-metal stents. JAMA 2006;295:1264.

[35] Rao SV, Shaw RE, Brindis RG, et al. Patterns and outcomes of drug-eluting coronary stent use in clinical practice. Am Heart J 2006;152:321.

[36] Joner M, Finn AV, Farb A, et al. Pathology of drug-eluting stents in humans: delayed healing and late thrombotic risk. J Am Coll Cardiol 2006;48:193.

[37] Applegate RJ, Sacrinty MT, Little WC, et al. Incidence of coronary stent thrombosis based on academic research consortium definitions. Am J Cardiol 2008;102:683.

[38] Zamanian R, Haddad F, Doyle RL, et al. Management strategies for patients with pulmonary hypertension in the intensive care unit. Crit Care Med 2007;35:2037.

[39] Goy JJ, Urban P, Kaufmann U, et al. Incidence of stent thrombosis and adverse cardiac events 5 years after sirolimus stent implantation in clinical practice. Am Heart J 2009;157:883.

[40] Roy P, Bonnello L, Torguson R, et al. Temporal relations between clopidogrel cessation and stent thrombosis after drug-eluting stent implantation. Am Cardiol 2009;103(6):801.

[41] Hao PP, Chen YG, Wang XL, et al. Efficacy and safety of drug-eluting stents in patients with acute ST-segment-elevation myocardial infarction: a meta-analysis of randomized controlled trials. Tex Heart Inst J 2010;37:516.

[42] Sibbing D, Steinhubl SR, Schulz S, et al. Platelet aggregation and its association with stent thrombosis and bleeding in clopidogrel-treated patients: initial evidence of a therapeutic window. J Am Coll Cardiol 2010;56:317.

[43] Capodanno D, Dipasqua F, Tamburino C. Novel drug-eluting stents in the treatment of de novo coronary lesions. Vasc Health Risk Manag 2011;7:103.

[44] Di Mario C, Ferrante G. Biodegradable drug-eluting stents: promises and pitfalls. Lancet 2008;371:873.

[45] Ormiston JA, Serruys PW, Regar E, et al. A bioabsorbable everolimus-eluting coronary stent system for patients with single de-novo coronary artery lesions (ABSORB): a prospective open-label trial. Lancet 2008;371:899.

[46] Norgard NB, Abu-Fadel M. Comparison of prasurgrel and clopidogrel in patients with acute coronary syndrome undergoing percutaneous coronary intervention. Vasc Health Risk Manag 2009;5:873.

[47] Beohar N, Davidson CJ, Kip KE, et al. Outcomes and complications associated with off-label and untested use of drug-eluting stents. JAMA 1992;297:2007.

[48] Baldwin DE, Abbott JD, Trost JC, et al. Comparison of drug-eluting and bare metal stents for saphenous vein graft lesions (from the National Heart, Lung, and Blood Institute Dynamic Registry). Am J Cardiol 2010;106:946.

[49] Nobuyoshi M, Kimura T, Nosaka H, et al. Restenosis after successful percutaneous transluminal coronary angioplasty: serial angiographic follow-up of 229 patients. J Am Coll Cardiol 1988;12:616.

[50] Popma JJ, Califf RM, Topol EJ. Clinical trials of restenosis after coronary angioplasty. Circulation 1991;84:1426.

[51] Allen JR, Helling TS, Hartzler GO. Operative procedures not involving the heart after percutaneous transluminal coronary angioplasty. Surg Gynecol Obstet 1991;173:258.

[52] Huber KC, Evans MA, Bresnahan JF, et al. Outcome of noncardiac operations in patients with severe coronary artery disease successfully treated preoperatively with coronary angioplasty. Mayo Clin Proc 1992;67:15.

[53] Gottlieb A, Banoub M, Sprung J, et al. Perioperative cardiovascular morbidity in patients with coronary artery disease undergoing vascular surgery after percutaneous transluminal coronary angioplasty. J Cardiothorac Vasc Anesth 1998;12:501.

[54] Brilakis ES, Orford JL, Fasseas P, et al. Outcome of patients undergoing balloon angioplasty in the two months prior to noncardiac surgery. Am J Cardiol 2005;96:512.

[55] Rabbitts J, Nuttall GA, Brown MJ, et al. Cardiac risk of noncardiac surgery after percutaneous coronary intervention with drug-eluting stents. Anesthesiology 2008;109:596.

[56] Eberli D, Chassot P-G, Sulser T, et al. Urological surgery and antiplatelet drugs after cardiac and cerebrovascular accidents. J Urol 2010;183:2128.

[57] Sharma AK, Ajani AE, Hamwi SM, et al. Major noncardiac surgery following coronary stenting: when is it safe to operate? Catheter Cardiovasc Interv 2004;63:141.

[58] Schouten O, van Domburg RT, Bax JJ, et al. Noncardiac surgery after coronary stenting: early surgery and interruption of antiplatelet therapy are associated with an increase in major adverse cardiac events. J Am Coll Cardiol 2007;49:122.

[59] McFalls EO, Ward HB, Moritz TE, et al. Coronary-artery revascularization before elective major vascular surgery. N Engl J Med 2004;351:2795.

[60] Poldermans D, Schouten O, Vidakovic R, et al. A clinical randomized trial to evaluate the safety of a noninvasive approach in high-risk patients undergoing major vascular surgery: the DECREASE-V Pilot Study. J Am Coll Cardiol 2007;49:1763.

[61] Hertzer NR, Young JR, Kramer JR, et al. Routine coronary angiography prior to elective aortic reconstruction: results of selective myocardial revascularization in patients with peripheral vascular disease. Arch Surg 1979;114:1336.

[62] Schouten O, van Kuijk JP, Flu WJ, et al. Long-term outcome of prophylactic coronary revascularization in cardiac high-risk patients undergoing major vascular surgery (from the Randomized DECREASE-V Pilot Study). Am J Cardiol 2009;103:897.

[63] Biccard BM, Rodseth RN. A meta-analysis of the prospective randomised trials of coronary revascularisation before noncardiac vascular surgery with attention to the type of coronary revascularisation performed. Anaesthesia 2009;64:1105.

[64] Steinhubl SR, Berger PB, Mann JT, et al. Early and sustained dual oral antiplatelet therapy following percutaneous coronary intervention. JAMA 2002;288:2411.

[65] Serebruany VL, Malinin AI, Ferguson JJ, et al. Bleeding risks of combination vs. single antiplatelet therapy: a meta-analysis of 18 randomized trials comprising 129,314 patients. Fundam Clin Pharmacol 2008;22:315.

[66] Purkayastha S, Athanasiou T, Malinovski V, et al. Does clopidogrel affect outcome after coronary artery bypass grafting? A meta-analysis. Heart 2006;92:531.

[67] Stone DH, Goodney PP, Schanzer A, et al. Clopidogrel is not associated with major bleeding complications during peripheral arterial surgery. J Vasc Surgery 2011. DOI:10.1016/j.jvs.2011.03.003.

[68] Ferraris VA, Swanson E. Aspirin usage and perioperative blood loss in patients undergoing unexpected surgery. Surg Gynecol Obstet 1983;156:439.

[69] Burger W, Chemnitius JM, Kneissl GD, et al. Low-dose aspirin for secondary cardiovascular prevention–cardiovascular risks after its perioperative withdrawal versus bleeding risks with its continuation–review and meta-analysis. J Intern Med 2005;257:399.

[70] Horlocker T, Wedel DJ, Schroeder DR, et al. Preoperative antiplatelet therapy does not increase the risk of spinal hematoma associated with regional anesthesia. Anesth Analg 1995;80:303.

[71] Savonitto S, D'Urbano M, Caracciolo M, et al. Urgent surgery in patients with a recently implanted coronary drug-eluting stent: a phase II study of 'bridging' antiplatelet therapy with tirofiban during temporary withdrawal of clopidogrel. Br J Anaesth 2010;104:285.

[72] Chechik O, Thein R, Fichman G, et al. The effect of clopidogrel and aspirin on blood loss in hip fracture surgery. Injury 2011. DOI:10.1016/j.injury.2011.01.011.

[73] Horlocker T, Wedel DJ, Rowlingson JC, et al. Executive summary: regional anesthesia in the patient receiving antithrombotic or thrombolytic therapy: American Society of Regional Anesthesia and Pain Medicine Evidence-Based Guidelines (Third Edition). Reg Anesth Pain Med 2010;35:102.

[74] Eikelboom JW, Hirsh J. Bleeding and management of bleeding. Eur Heart J Suppl 2006;8:G38.

[75] Gurbel PA, Tantry US. Combination antithrombotic therapies. Circulation 2010;121:569.

[76] Wiviott SD, Antman EM, Braunwald E. Prasugrel. Circulation 2010;122:394.

[77] Gurbel PA, Antonino MJ, Tantry US. Recent developments in clopidogrel pharmacology and their relation to clinical outcomes. Expert Opin Drug Metab Toxicol 2009;5:989.

[78] Wiviott SD, Antman EM, Winters KJ, et al. Randomized comparison of prasugrel (CS-747, LY640315), a novel thienopyridine P2Y12 antagonist, with clopidogrel in percutaneous coronary intervention: results of the Joint Utilization of Medications to Block Platelets Optimally (JUMBO)-TIMI 26 trial. Circulation 2005;111:3366.

[79] Inhibition of platelet glycoprotein IIb/IIIa with eptifibatide in patients with acute coronary syndromes. N Engl J Med 1998;339:436.

[80] Inhibition of the platelet glycoprotein IIb/IIIa receptor with tirofiban in unstable angina and non-Q-wave myocardial infarction. N Engl J Med 1998;338:1488.

[81] von Segesser LK, Killer I, Ziswiler M, et al. Dissection of the descending thoracic aorta extending into the ascending aorta—a therapeutic challenge. J Thorac Cardiovasc Surg 1994;108:755.

[82] Perkins WJ, Lanzino G, Brott TG. Carotid stenting vs endarterectomy: new results in perspective. Mayo Clin Proc 2010;85:1101.

[83] Randomised trial of endarterectomy for recently symptomatic carotid stenosis: final results of the MRC European Carotid Surgery Trial (ECST). Lancet 1998;351:1379.

[84] Beneficial effect of carotid endarterectomy in symptomatic patients with high-grade carotid stenosis. N Engl J Med 1991;325:445.

[85] Barnett HJ, Taylor DW, Eliasziw M, et al. Benefit of carotid endarterectomy in patients with symptomatic moderate or severe stenosis. N Engl J Med 1998;339:1415.

[86] Hobson RW, Weiss DG, Fields WS, et al. Efficacy of carotid endarterectomy for asymptomatic carotid stenosis. N Engl J Med 1993;328:221.

[87] National Institute of Neurological Disorders, Walker MD, Marler JR, Goldstein M, et al. Executive Committee for the Asymptomatic Carotid Atherosclerosis Study. endarterectomy for asymptomatic carotid artery stenosis. JAMA 1995;273:1421.

[88] Prevention of disabling and fatal strokes by successful carotid endarterectomy in patients without recent neurological symptoms: randomised controlled trial. Lancet 2004;363:1491.

[89] Sacco RL, Adams R, Albers G, et al. Guidelines for prevention of stroke in patients with ischemic stroke or transient ischemic attack: a statement for healthcare professionals from the American Heart Association/American Stroke Association Council on stroke: co-sponsored by the Council on Cardiovascular Radiology and Intervention: the American Academy of Neurology affirms the value of this guideline. Circulation 2006;113:e409.

[90] Howell GM, Makaroun MS, Chaer RA. Current management of extracranial carotid occlusive disease. J Am Coll Surg 2009;208:442.

[91] Adams HP. Secondary prevention of atherothrombotic events after ischemic stroke. Mayo Clin Proc 2009;84:43.

[92] Lanzino G, Rabinstein AA, Brown RD. Treatment of carotid artery stenosis: medical therapy, surgery, or stenting? Mayo Clin Proc 2009;84:362.

[93] Marsh JD, Keyrouz SG. Stroke prevention and treatment. J Am Coll Cardiol 2010;56:683.

[94] Wu T, Grotta JC. Stroke treatment and prevention: five new things. Neurology 2010;75(18 Suppl 1):S16.

[95] van der Vaart MG, Meerwaldt R, Reijnen MM, et al. Endarterectomy or carotid artery stenting: the quest continues. Am J Surg 2008;195:259.

[96] Hassoun HT, Malas MB, Freischlag JA. Secondary stroke prevention in the era of carotid stenting: update on recent trials. Arch Surg 2010;145:928.

[97] Carotid artery stenting compared with endarterectomy in patients with symptomatic carotid stenosis (International Carotid Stenting Study): an interim analysis of a randomised controlled trial. Lancet 2010;375:985.

[98] Brott TG, Hobson RW, Howard G, et al. Stenting versus endarterectomy for treatment of carotid-artery stenosis. N Engl J Med 2010;363:11.

[99] Meier P, Knapp G, Tamhane U, et al. Short term and intermediate term comparison of endarterectomy versus stenting for carotid artery stenosis: systematic review and meta-analysis of randomised controlled clinical trials. BMJ 2010;340:c467.

[100] Buhk J, Wellmer A, Knauth M, et al. Late in-stent thrombosis following carotid angioplasty and stenting. Neurology 2010;66:1594.

[101] Perera GB, Lyden SP. Current trends in lower extremity revascularization. Surg Clin North Am 2007;87:1135.

[102] White CJ, Gray WA. Endovascular therapies for peripheral arterial disease: an evidence-based review. Circulation 2007;116:2203.

[103] White CJ. Management of renal artery stenosis: the case for intervention, defending current guidelines, and screening (drive-by) renal angiography at the time of catheterization. Prog Cardiovasc Dis 2009;52:229.

[104] Dworkin LD, Cooper CJ. Renal-artery stenosis. N Engl J Med 2009;361:1972.

Advances in Anesthesia 29 (2011) 113–127

ADVANCES IN ANESTHESIA

ELSEVIER
MOSBY

Drug Diversion, Chemical Dependence, and Anesthesiology

John E. Tetzlaff, MD

Department of General Anesthesia, Anesthesiology Institute, Cleveland Clinic Lerner College of Medicine of Case Western Reserve University, Cleveland Clinic, 9500 Euclid Avenue, E31, Cleveland, OH 44195, USA

The "tools of the trade" for those who give anesthesia are potent drugs. Mastery of their use is an essential element of the specialty. By the nature of clinical practice in the operating room (OR), the anesthesia provider is continuously obtaining, using, and accounting for controlled substances in considerable quantities. The process makes the provider an expert in parenteral administration of substances. In addition to facilitating the administration of anesthesia, this repetitive process creates ideal conditions for diversion of controlled substances and self-medication. The unfortunate reality is that self-medication rapidly and reliably leads to chemical dependency with an unusually high potential for morbidity and mortality. Despite a heightened level of awareness, education about risk, and other efforts to prevent diversion, the incidence remains uncomfortably high. The result is that addiction to anesthesia drugs with its consequences is the leading cause of death in young anesthesia providers.

SCOPE OF THE PROBLEM

The United States is known to be the "addiction capital of the world" (Box 1). Addiction to anesthesia drugs by anesthesia providers is one unique subcategory of this phenomenon, although it is not confined to the United States. Addiction to anesthesia drugs has been reported essentially as long as the drugs have been known to have a human use. Recreational use of cocaine and opiates has hundreds, even thousands, of years of history. Soon after the properties of nitrous oxide and ether were discovered and demonstrated, illicit use was reported. Some of this can be attributed to the nineteenth-century axiom of science: "a good scientist always tries it on himself first."

As anesthesia began to evolve into a unique medical specialty in the mid-twentieth century, data began to accumulate about the people who chose the

The author has nothing to disclose.

E-mail address: tetzlaj@ccf.org

0737-6146/11/$ – see front matter
doi:10.1016/j.aan.2011.07.004

Box 1: Scope of the problem

The United States has a high prevalence of substance use and is thought to have the highest per-person rate of substance abuse in the world

- 160 million Americans use caffeine
- 60 million tobacco/nicotine users
- 18 million alcoholics
- 6 million users of illicit substances
- 1–3 million with physical dependence

specialty. Because clinical practice of anesthesia involved frequent exposure to potent chemicals (ether, chloroform, cyclopropane, halothane), there was concern about chronic organ toxicity and shortened life span. In data from two studies spanning almost 30 years (1947–1976), longevity of physicians practicing anesthesia was average, with no peaks of heart, lung, liver, kidney disease, or cancer, but with a notably high incidence of accidents and suicide as causes of death [1,2]. Young male anesthesiologists (age 25–34 years) had 3.4 times the age-adjusted suicide rate compared with other physicians [1]. Many of the "accidents" undoubtedly were related to addiction [2]. Although much of the data and publicity originates from the United States, the same addiction pattern has been reported in the United Kingdom [3] as well as Australia and New Zealand [4].

Because the incidence seems so high and the consequences so serious, there have been numerous, well-subscribed surveys to determine the incidence. Ward and colleagues [5] collected data for the 1970s and reported an incidence of 1% per year in the first 5 years of giving anesthesia. Gravenstein and colleagues [6] also reported a 1% per year incidence with a disturbing mortality of 7 of 44 addicted residents. Booth and colleagues [7] reported incidences of 1.6% per year in residency and 1.0% per year for junior staff between 1985 and 1995. Collins and colleagues [8] reported data from 1991 to 2001, with 80% of programs who responded reporting one incident or more, and 19% reporting at least one mortality. Despite substantial increases in education and tighter regulation of controlled substances [7], the incidence seems to be increasing, as is the associated morbidity [8].

DEMOGRAPHICS OF PROVIDERS WITH CHEMICAL DEPENDENCY

When all available data are reviewed, it is clear that every category of provider has been involved in this epidemic of addiction to anesthesia drugs. Although most obvious in allopathic physicians because of sheer numbers, it has been reported with a comparable incidence in the osteopathic anesthesia community [8]. The risk for the Certified Registered Nurse Anesthetist (CRNA) and Student Registered Nurse Anesthetist (SRNA) categories is the same or higher [9–11]. Addiction has been reported in Anesthesia Assistants and Oral Surgeons with anesthesia training in direct proportion to the time spent in anesthesia training [12].

Other characteristics that cross provider categories are a young age range and high academic performance. The peak in young individuals is related to the observation that addiction occurs most frequently in the first 5 years of giving anesthesia. This finding has been reported for residents [5,13], SRNAs/CRNAs [11], and Oral Surgeons [12]. From the American Society of Anesthesiologists (ASA) database, it is evident that some of the most academically talented people in the specialty (AOA, Phi Beta Kappa) are among those found to be addicted. A similar peak in the upper 10% of SRNA Classes is found [11].

One other element that all categories of providers have in common is the devastating consequences of this addiction pattern to individuals, careers, families, and departments. The progression is very rapid [14], occurs in individuals new to the specialty [11,13], creates serious disability [3], and is associated with high morbidity and mortality [5,6,8,15]. Often the first manifestation of chemical dependency is coma, accidental death, or suicide [5,16].

WHY DOES ADDICTION PLAGUE THOSE WHO PRACTICE ANESTHESIA?

Much has been written about the causes for self-medication, chemical dependency, and the morbidity associated with addiction to anesthesia substances. One universal consensus is that this syndrome has multifactorial causes (Box 2), but the data supporting conclusions about this issue range from expert opinion, to inference, to pure speculation.

There has been a lot of speculation about characteristics of individuals before entry into medicine and/or anesthesia that predict, or are associated with, subsequent self-medication with anesthetic drugs. One element that has widespread

---

Box 2: Risk factors for addiction to anesthesia drugs

- Long work hours
- Isolation
- Stress
- "The chemical solution"
- Availability of drugs
- Direct observation of drug actions
- Denial
- Prolonged delayed gratification within the physician personality
- The "omnipotence" of physicians
- Economic resources to purchase

agreement from the experts is prior chemical experimentation. In a large survey of medical students, a substantial number admitted to chemical experimentation [17]. Experts in anesthesia addiction are convinced that prior experimentation is associated with subsequent chemical dependency to anesthesia drugs, based on interviews with patients in rehabilitation [8,18]. This finding is consistent with another observation from the psychiatry literature, namely, that high-risk behavior of all kinds correlates with subsequent addictive behavior [19].

Additional agreement among addiction experts supports that coexisting psychiatric illness is associated with addiction. "Abnormal" behavior has been reported in a substantial number (10%–20%) of surveyed medical students [20]. A prior history of psychiatric illness has been observed in a majority of addicted anesthesia providers in interviews conducted during rehabilitation [13,19–21]. There is a particularly high association of personality disorders in addicted physicians [22]. Speculation based on observation suggests that self-medication may be a symptom of depression, and could explain the association of depression with addiction [23].

An intriguing hypothesis to explain this serious occupational hazard is that addiction to anesthetic drugs is caused by handling of the substances. Much of the data is highly speculative. As mentioned previously, experimenting with new potential anesthetic drugs in the nineteenth century not only led to knowledge about their efficacy but also to addiction of the investigators. Also previously mentioned is the observation that addiction often occurs in the first 5 years of exposure to giving anesthesia [5,11–13] in all categories of providers. Although this does not prove that handling is cause for addiction, it certainly is highly suggestive when individuals become chemically dependent on drugs they have just begun to handle. Further support for this speculation comes from the work of Gold and colleagues [14], who have verified that there is measurable chronic exposure to a variety of anesthesia drugs related to the preparation to administer the drugs (eg, fentanyl, propofol), and via exhaled breath of patients during emergence from anesthesia [24]. These observations led Gold and colleagues [14] to speculate that chronic exposure to anesthesia drugs leads a subset of anesthesia providers to be neurochemically predisposed to self-medicate. These observations were challenged by the ASA Committee on Occupational Health because many of the conclusions were based on speculation, and because of the implications for the specialty [25]. However, there is evidence in animals that chronic exposure to opioids activates brain reward centers, leading to addictive behavior [26]. Further speculation originates from increasing information about molecular mechanisms of addiction. It is clear that exposure to addictive drugs results in electron transfer, creating reactive oxygen species (free radicals that activate brain reward centers), predisposing the individual to further self-medication with the same substance, and to subsequent addiction [27]. More recent information confirms that exposure to fentanyl or propofol creates these same molecular messengers [28].

Elements of anesthesia practice probably produce some of the urge to self-medicate. Farley and Talbott [29] list some of these elements, including long work hours, extended intervals of being alone creating feelings of isolation, and personal belief in the "chemical solution" (which may have played a role in the individual choosing the specialty). Health care providers are often drawn to anesthesia in part by interest in pharmacology, and the clinical observation that there are drugs to adjust almost every human parameter. This love of the "chemical solution" may also predispose providers to self-medicate. In addition, the comprehensive handling of controlled substances is almost surely a factor. Anesthesia team members are the only individuals in the health care team who decide to medicate, and then with their own hands obtain the substance, draw it up, administer it, observe the consequences, chart the administration, and document the wastage. From the very beginning of anesthesia training, the anesthesia provider learns very quickly the clinical dose/response information for analgesic and sedative drugs. Another skill that is rapidly acquired is accurate and technically correct parenteral administration of substances, a skill that is unfortunately ideal training for self-medication. This training for self-medication occurs in the environment of the OR. The OR environment is hard on beginners, with stress, production pressure, self-esteem issues reinforced by implied hierarchy, and the uncertainty of a new environment. This scenario is particularly relevant in the context of the data previously presented that self-medication can be a symptom of depression [23]. The natural curiosity about drugs, combined with the stress that is inevitable during anesthesia training, undoubtedly causes some to make unfortunate choices.

THE CHEMICAL PROFILE

The chemical profile of anesthesia drugs diverted for addiction correlates with the dates of training. Before 1980, the most common drugs diverted for self-medication were meperidine, diazepam, and barbiturates [30,31]. After 1980, the vast majority of chemical dependency in anesthesia providers has involved drugs in the fentanyl family [5,7,12,29]. At a much lower incidence, there are reports of diversion and self-medication with other substances, including nitrous oxide [32], ketamine [33], midazolam [12] and potent inhalation agents [34]. Although the incidence of self-medication with potent inhalation agents seems low, a survey of academic departments revealed a large number (22% of those responding) reporting at least one incident with poor outcome, and a high overall level of morbidity [35]. Propofol is playing an increasingly prominent role in chemical dependency for anesthesia providers. A case report detailed repeated self-injection to the point of unconsciousness numerous times daily over an extended period [36]. In response to the apparent increase in propofol diversion, a survey revealed that 18% of residency programs had one incident, and 7 deaths were reported for the period from 1995 to 2005 [15]. Over 10 years, propofol abuse has evolved from episodic case reports of self-medication to a rate estimated at 10% of the incidence of fentanyl addiction, and most experts believe the rate of propofol abuse is increasing further [15]. The seriousness of the issue with propofol is receiving increasing scrutiny by national organizations. The Drug Enforcement Administration (DEA) of the

Department of Justice has begun to review the status of propofol as an uncontrolled substance. Their review of the abuse potential for propofol, reported cases, and the fact that a chemically similar drug, fospropofol, was released onto the market as a schedule IV controlled substance, has led the DEA to publish a proposed rule (21 CFR Part 1308), which would make propofol a schedule IV controlled substance. This proposed rule was published in the Federal Register (75 Fed. Reg 66196) on October 27, 2010. Because of the impact on clinical practice this rule was published with an interval for comment, which continues at the time of this writing. The ASA and the American Association of Nurse Anesthetists have both issued position papers and formal DEA comments strongly supporting implementation of this rule. Given the increasing incidence and the known morbidity associated with the self-medication of propofol [15], moving propofol to controlled substance status would seem both rational and inevitable.

The abuse potential for fentanyl lies in the euphoria and anxiolysis that occurs rapidly and predictably. With propofol, anxiolysis occurs very rapidly, and has been reported to be associated with erotic imaging in some individuals. Intoxication is reported by those who self-medicate with potent inhalation agents. Among the drugs less frequently diverted by anesthesia providers, the abuse potential can be predicted from the side-effect profile, such as cocaine (euphoria), antihistamines (sedation), local anesthetics (dysphoria), and ephedrine (stimulation). In this same frame of reference, abuse of ketamine highly correlates with prior illicit exposure to psychotropic drugs [33,37].

The characteristics of anesthetic drugs predict their abuse potential and its consequences. The combination of familiarity and skill with administration lead to what Farley and Talbott [29] called the "fallacy of control." The individual under stress identifies a chemical solution (self-medication), and the learned skill with the use of the substance possessed by the provider leads them to the false conclusion that they can control the consequences of self-medication. In one extreme case, a single experiment with intranasal application of sufentanil evolved into 30 mL per day being injected within 30 days [14]. Ward and colleagues [5] summarized the opinion of experts that an individual who self-medicates with a member of the fentanyl family is addicted after the first attempt, even if they do not recognize it at that time. Feedback from individuals in rehabilitation supports this belief.

HOW DOES CHEMICAL DEPENDENCY IN ANESTHESIA PROVIDERS REVEAL ITSELF?

Although the signs of addiction in anesthesia providers are well known (Box 3), they are often initially subtle and hard to distinguish from fatigue, stress, or other common life events. When self-medication with anesthetic drugs is sustained, it rapidly accelerates. At present the level of awareness of the inevitable consequences of fentanyl addiction are widely known, and most individuals reveal in rehabilitation that they were well aware of the deadly consequences. However, self-reporting is unusual and, in fact, coma, suicide, and accidental

Box 3: Recognizing substance abuse in anesthesia providers

Self-reporting or seeking help is unfortunately very uncommon among anesthesia providers. Recognition of a problem often depends on the observations of peers or family. Signs include:

- Behavior changes
- Clinical performance changes
- Inappropriate behavior
- Mood swings
- Decreased attention to appearance or hygiene
- Drowsiness
- Urgent requests for breaks
- Issues with handling of controlled substances
- Lethargy
- Unusual financial problems
- Social embarrassment (extreme behavior)
- Legal conflict (driving under the influence and so forth)
- Sloppy medical records
- New skin problems
- Regular wearing of gowns, long-sleeve shirts
- Frequent requests to work extra nights or weekend calls
- Falling asleep in the OR

death are more common than self-reporting [29]. The most common trigger for detection is observed abnormal behavior, which triggers an audit, confirming diversion. A promising new approach to detection driven by electronic records is the creation of user profiles designed to flag outliers [38].

Confirmation of self-medication is difficult at best. Most of the preferred drugs of abuse are difficult to detect because of short metabolic half-lives or nondetectable substances [39,40]. A promising new option for detection of propofol is an assay for the propofol glucuronide metabolites, which are present in the urine for up to 72 hours. When typical Emergency Department algorithms are used to perform "for cause" testing, urine toxicology can fail in relation to timing, because the drugs of abuse common in the lay public have longer half-lives [41]. Audits of drug use are also not foolproof, because of the compliance failures with accounting for controlled substance wastage that can exceed 10% of total cases in large medical centers [42]. A promising new approach, developed for confirmation of driving under the influence, is the use of rapid oral fluid testing [43]. Unfortunately, most anesthetic drugs of abuse cannot be detected by oral fluid testing at this time. The frustration with negative urine screening is evident in one case series where "for cause" screening was used based on suspicion, and was found to be repeatedly negative [44]. In each case, hair analysis revealed evidence of chronic exposure to fentanyl, sufentanil, and/or alfentanil. Unfortunately, hair analysis is difficult, requires a considerable volume of hair, and does not detect acute exposure [41]. The problems with confirmation of urine, blood, and hair toxicology are further compounded by the hundreds of options to mask substances in a urine-screening test [45]. Clean urine, realistic-appearing urogenital facades, and agent-specific blocking agents for illicit drugs can be purchased via the Internet [46]. Even preemployment testing has an unclear impact on the incidence of subsequent addiction, and still needs data-driven review to determine its value [47]. Preemployment screening will have no impact on the incidence of chemical dependency in anesthesiology unless the anesthetic drugs are part of the screening (Box 4). Routine urine toxicology focuses on illicit drugs and does not identify fentanil, propofol, ketamine, and so forth. The specific testing panels for random testing (Box 5) and "for cause" testing (Box 6) must be specifically requested from the testing laboratory because urine screening in the vast majority of instances does not seek any of the anesthesia drugs, and the cost differential per test is considerable for adding these drugs to the screening profile. Sophisticated user profiles linked to electronic anesthesia and pharmacy records has great potential in the future [38]. At a minimum, these tools should improve the options to investigate discrepancies in the reporting between drug withdrawal and use/wastage accounting.

CAREER DISPOSITION AFTER REHABILITATION OF CHEMICAL DEPENDENCY TO ANESTHESIA DRUGS

Although the risk of reentry (relapse, death) is known and failures are associated with a high level of morbidity, the majority of addicted anesthesia providers ask to reenter anesthesia when released from inpatient treatment,

---

Box 4: Screening panel for preemployment of anesthesia providers

"Preemployment" testing will screen for:
- Amphetamines
- Barbiturates
- Benzodiazepines
- Cocaine
- Methadone
- Opiates
- Opioids (fentanyl family)
- Phencyclidine
- Propoxyphene
- Marijuana
- Propofol Glucuronide

Box 5: Screening panel for random testing of anesthesia providers

The profile for "random" testing will include:

- Opiates
- Opioids (fentanyl family)
- Methadone
- Morphine
- Meperidine
- Heroin
- Dilaudid
- Midazolam/diazepam
- Propoxyphene
- Cocaine
- Propofol glucuronide

Box 6: Screening panel to be used in "for cause" testing of anesthesia providers

When "for cause" testing is indicated, the substances screened will include:

- Amphetamines
- Barbiturates
- Benzodiazepines
- Cocaine
- Marijuana
- Methadone
- Morphine
- Meperidine
- Opiates
- Opioids
- Phencyclidine
- Heroin
- Dilaudid
- Midazolam/diazepam
- Propoxyphene
- Fentanyl
- Propofol Glucuronide
- Ketamine
- Ethylene hydroxide (breath alcohol test [BAT])

this despite the increasing body of evidence suggesting that giving anesthesia is associated with relapse, and that relapse has a high mortality rate. There are several issues.

First, addiction is a disease and its consequences are considered a federally protected disability (Americans with Disability Act) as long as the individual is in compliance with an ongoing treatment plan [48]. Addicted providers will often respond to advice to change specialties by countering with the argument that their disability is protected and reentry is a right. There is no clear evidence of patient risk, although it should be noted that case law has become progressively less protective of the addicted physician [48].

Evidence regarding the outcome of reentry for providers with chemical dependency to anesthetic drugs is variable, but appears generally discouraging. Physicians appear to have better outcomes from rehabilitation than the general public [49]. Specifically, physicians have better outcomes after rehabilitation for prescription opiate abuse compared with the lay public [50]. There is some evidence that this favorable outcome also applies to physicians with addiction to anesthetic drugs [51], although in some reports the definition of success may be generous, allowing for up to 2 relapses [52,53]. Aggressive participation of state physician health programs seems to improve the outcome of reentry [51].

Despite the aforementioned, there is an increasing body of evidence that reentry has a low success rate and high level of risk. Collins and colleagues [8] report that more than 40% of residents who reenter anesthesiology residency do not complete their training, have a very high relapse rate, and a 9% mortality. Merk and colleagues [54] reported a series of failures of reentry, with the first indication of relapse being death in 16%. Reentry for student nurse anesthetists is equally unsuccessful and risky [10]. Bryson and Levine [55] reported an innovative program for reentry in an academic center. The individual undergoes inpatient treatment, and on release to work they become faculty for an anesthesia simulation center. This program allows activity within the anesthesia world, gainful employment, contact with the anesthesia team, and a schedule that allows outpatient care to continue. Their protocol allows for this status to continue for 12 to 18 months, until the treatment team determines that return to clinical anesthesia is indicated. Despite this generous, resource-demanding protocol, they report a 60% relapse rate in the first 5 patients. Other investigators [56] have formed the opinion that reentry should be denied and retraining in another specialty should be universally applied ("one strike and you're out"). Another approach is rigidly structured reentry, with delayed assignment to on-call responsibility, another provider handling all controlled drugs, mandatory meetings, and toxicology screening, all managed by a written contract with state physician health programs [57].

When treatment of chemical dependency is directed toward reentry, the conduct of the rehabilitation program must adapt. Hedberg [58] makes it clear there are risks with reentry, and that the decision to allow return to clinical anesthesia must be made by the treatment team and not be overly influenced by the patient or the sponsoring department. Hedberg also identifies several elements that he believes should either delay reentry or require the treatment team to recommend against reentry. This standpoint is a serious one, because compliance with the treatment plan is a condition of disability protection. Further review of the reentry data identifies several independent factors that are associated with failure, including unresolved psychiatric disorders, family history of substance abuse, or long addiction (>1 year) to opioids [59].

STRATEGIES TO REDUCE THE INCIDENCE OF CHEMICAL DEPENDENCE ON ANESTHESIA DRUGS

For more than 30 years, it has been known that addiction to anesthesia drugs is an occupational safety hazard for those who administer anesthesia. Education in substance abuse has become a universal part of anesthesia training, but there has been no decline in the incidence of abuse despite substantial increases in education and awareness [7]. There has also been attention directed to issues of wellness that contribute to addiction, including stress management and fatigue. It will be interesting, when the data become known, to examine the impact of the Accreditation Council for Graduate Medical Education restrictions on duty hours for anesthesiology residents with addictive disease. Booth and colleagues [7] argue that education fails because staff are not included, reexposure to the topic after residency is uncommon, and families are not included, even though addiction is, in so many respects, a family disease. Many of these defects in education have been acknowledged and education has broadly increased, but still the result has been no corresponding decrease in the incidence of addicted providers [60].

Another element in the strategy to decrease chemical dependency is to specifically target and reduce diversion of controlled substances by anesthesia providers. Recognition of this problem has led departments to expend and increase time and resources to prevent diversion, including video surveillance, lock boxes, satellite pharmacies, random screening of waste syringes, and electronic dispensing systems [7,61]. In the report by Booth and colleagues [7], 60% of departments reported substantially increasing their security for handling controlled drugs, again with no impact on the incidence of division. An insight into this contradiction can be found in the report of Vigoda and colleagues [42], revealing a greater than 10% discrepancy between the electronic anesthetic record and the electronic drug dispensing record. Electronic screening [62] and user profiles [38] may have a role in prevention, as well as the role in detection previously mentioned.

The use of urine toxicology for prevention and early detection is controversial. The American Medical Association (AMA) advocates only preemployment and "for cause" testing because of concerns about confidentiality and bias in selection for random testing [63,64]. When polled, the majority of anesthesia chairs favored random testing [7], although few have implemented programs after preemployment testing. Random urine testing is universally applied within the military, the Department of Transportation (DOT), and in a majority of companies in the United States with greater than 5000 employees [65]. Review of industrial application of random screening suggests that it reduces health care–related costs [66]. The position of the ASA was expressed by its previous legal advisor, Mike Scott [67], who identified the legal risk with "for cause" (none), preemployment (minimal), and random (considerable) urine screening in the anesthesia context. The legal risk with random testing is reduced by the "safety exception," which generally allows for random testing in jobs where the public safety is involved. Anesthesia has been defined as included in this "safety exception" in several legal cases. Concern of the AMA about bias and false positives are actually addressed in the DOT protocols for random testing. The DOT rules define the role of the Medical Review Officer in generating random lists and determining true positives by eliminating false positives related to legitimate medical explanations for substances in the urine [68]. A report of the first 5 years of random screening in the Massachusetts General Hospital anesthesia department revealed no true positives [69]. Failure to intervene with providers showing evident impairment has demonstrated legal risk [70], whereas an intervention to confront the individual and force treatment, even incomplete with a bad outcome (total denial by the addict), does not subject the intervention team to legal risk [71].

SUMMARY

Chemical dependence on anesthesia drugs is the most significant occupational safety hazard associated with administering anesthesia. The consequences are serious for career, family, and the department. The incidence is uncomfortably high, peaks at the beginning of careers, and is increasingly well known to the lay public. Evidence is highly suggestive that handling of anesthesia drugs is causative, as are some of the conditions associated with anesthesia practice (self-esteem issues, isolation, production pressure, stress, and so forth). Return to practice after treatment for addiction to anesthesia drugs is controversial because of common failure and high mortality or morbidity. Education and security in handling of controlled substances has increased, but the incidence of chemical dependency has not. Prevention by electronic screening and random testing would seem to be trends for the future.

References

[1] Bruce DL, Eide KA, Linde HW, et al. Cause of death among anesthesiologists. Anesthesiology 1968;29:565–9.

[2] Lew EA. Mortality experience among anesthesiologists. Anesthesiology 1979;51:195–9.

[3] Berry CB, Crome IB, Plant M, et al. Substance misuse amongst anaesthetists in the United Kingdom and Ireland. Anaesthesia 2000;55:946–52.

[4] Weeks AM, Buckland MR, Morgan EB, et al. Chemical dependence in anaesthetic registrars in Australia and New Zealand. Anaesth Intensive Care 1993;21:151–5.

[5] Ward CF, Ward GC, Saidman LJ. Drug abuse in anesthesiology training programs. JAMA 1983;250:992–5.

[6] Gravenstein JS, Kory WP, Marks RG. Drug abuse by anesthesia personnel. Anesth Analg 1983;62:467–72.

[7] Booth JV, Grossman D, Moore J, et al. Substance abuse among physicians: a survey of academic anesthesiology programs. Anesth Analg 2002;95:1024–30.

[8] Collins GB, McAllister MS, Jensen M, et al. Chemical dependency treatment outcomes of residents in anesthesiology: results of a survey. Anesth Analg 2005;101:1457–62.

[9] Bell DM, McDonough JP, Ellison JS, et al. Controlled drug misuse by certified registered nurse anesthetists. AANA J 1999;67:133–40.

[10] Luck S, Hendrick J. The alarming trend of substance abuse in anesthesia providers. J Perianesth Nurs 2004;19:308–11.

[11] Clark GD, Stone JA. Assessment of the substance abuse curriculum in schools of nurse anesthesia. J Addiction Nursing 1999;11:123–35.

[12] Rosenberg M. Drug abuse in oral and maxillofacial training programs. J Oral Maxillofac Surg 1986;44:458–62.

[13] Talbott GD, Gallegos KV, Wilson PO, et al. The medical association of Georgia's impaired physician program: review of the first 1000 physicians. Analysis by specialty. JAMA 1987;257:2927–33.

[14] Gold MS, Byars JA, Frost-Pineda K. Occupational exposure and addictions for physicians: case studies and theoretical implications. Psychiatr Clin North Am 2004;27:745–53.

[15] Wischmeyer PE, Johnson BR, Wilson JE, et al. A survey of propofol abuse in academic anesthesia programs. Anesth Analg 2007;105:1066–71.

[16] Crawshaw R, Bruce JA, Eraker PL, et al. An epidemic of suicide among physicians on probation. JAMA 1980;243:1915–7.

[17] Epstein R, Eubanks EE. Drug use among medical students. N Engl J Med 1984;311:923.

[18] Gallegos KV, Browne LH, Veit FW, et al. Addiction in anesthesiologists: drug access and patterns of substance abuse. QRB Qual Rev Bull 1988;14(4):16–22.

[19] Yarborough WH. Substance use disorders in physician training programs. J Okla State Med Assoc 1999;92:504–7.

[20] Flaherty JA, Richman JA. Substance use and addiction among medical students, residents and physicians. Psychiatr Clin North Am 1993;16:189–97.

[21] Udel MM. Chemical abuse/dependence: physician's occupational hazard. J Med Assoc Ga 1984;73:775–8.

[22] Nance EP, Davis CW, Gaspart JP. Axis II co-morbidity in substance abusers. Am J Psychiatr 1991;148:118–20.

[23] Markov A, Kosten TR, Koob GF. Neurobiological similarities in depression and drug dependence: a self-medication hypothesis. Neuropharmacology 1998;18:135–74.

[24] Gold MS, Melker RJ, Dennis DM, et al. Fentanyl abuse and dependence: further evidence for the second hand exposure hypothesis. J Addict Dis 2006;25:15–21.

[25] Polk SL, Katz JD, Berry AJ, et al. Does ambient fentanyl enhance the susceptibility of anesthesiologists to addiction. ASA Newsl 2007;71:18–9.

[26] Mohar AR, Yao WD, Caron MG. Genetic and genomic approaches to reward and addiction. Neuropharmacology 2004;47:100–10.

[27] Kovacic P, Cooksy AL. Unifying mechanism for toxicity and addicting by abused drugs: electron transfer and reactive oxygen species. Med Hypotheses 2005;64:357–66.

[28] Kovacic P. Unifying electron transfer mechanism for addiction involvement by the anesthetic propofol. Med Hypotheses 2010;74:206.

[29] Farley WJ, Talbott GD. Anesthesiology and addiction. Anesth Analg 1983;62:465–6.

[30] Hughes PH, Brandenberg N, Baldwin DC, et al. Prevalence of substance use among US physicians. JAMA 1992;267:2333–9.

[31] Hughes PH, Baldwin DC, Sheehan DV, et al. Resident physician substance use by specialty. Am J Psychiatry 1992;149:1348–54.

[32] Suruda AJ, McGlothlin JD. Fatal abuse of nitrous oxide in the workplace. J Occup Med 1990;32:682–4.

[33] Moore NN, Bostwick JM. Ketamine dependence in anesthesia providers. Psychosomatics 1999;40:35609.

[34] Musshoff F, Junker H, Madea B. An unusual case of driving under the influence of enflurane. Forensic Sci Int 2002;128:18709.

[35] Wilson JE, Kiselanova N, Stevens Q, et al. A survey of inhalational anaesthetic abuse in anesthesia programmes. Anaesthesia 2008;63:616–20.

[36] Zacny JP, Lichtor JL, Thompson W, et al. Propofol at subanesthetic dose may have abuse potential in healthy volunteers. Anesth Analg 1993;77:544–52.

[37] Dalgarno PJ, Shewan D. Illicit use of ketamine in Scotland. J Psychoactive Drugs 1996;28: 191–9.

[38] Epstein RH. Development of a scheduled drug diversion surveillance system based on an analysis of atypical drug transactions. Anesth Analg 2007;105:1053–60.

[39] Hays LR, Stillner V, Littrell R. Fentanyl dependence associated with oral ingestion. Anesthesiology 1992;77:819–20.

[40] Henderson GL. The fentanyls. Am Assoc Clin Chem 1990;12:7–14.

[41] Verstraete AG. Detection times of drugs of abuse in blood, urine and oral fluid. Ther Drug Monit 2004;26:200–5.

[42] Vigoda MM, Gencorelli FJ, Lubarsky DA. Discrepancies in medication entries between anesthetic and pharmacy records using electronic databases. Anesth Analg 2007;105: 1061–5.

[43] Pil K, Vertraete A. Current developments in drug testing in oral fluid. Ther Drug Monit 2008;30:196–2000.

[44] Kintz P, Villain M, Dumestre V, et al. Evidence of addiction by anesthesiologists as documented by hair analysis. Forensic Sci Int 2005;153:81–4.

[45] Dasgusta A. The effects of adulterants and selected ingested compounds on drugs-of-abuse testing in urine. Am J Clin Pathol 2007;128:491–503.

[46] Jaffee WB, Trucco E, Levy S, et al. Is this urine really negative? A systematic review of tampering methods in urine drug screening and testing. J Subst Abuse Treat 2007;33: 33–42.

[47] Levine MR, Rennie WP. Pre-employment urine drug testing of hospital employees: future questions and review of current literature. Occup Environ Med 2004;61:318–24.

[48] Bryson EO, Silverstein JH. Addiction and substance abuse in anesthesiology. Anesthesiology 2008;109:905–17.

[49] Morse RM, Martin MA, Swenson WM, et al. Prognosis of physicians treated for alcoholism and drug dependence. JAMA 1984;251:743–6.

[50] Merlo LJ, Gold MS. Prescription opioid abuse and dependency among physicians; hypothesis and treatment. Harv Rev Psychiatry 2008;16:181–94.

[51] Skipper GE, Campbell MD, DuPont RL. Anesthesiologists with substance use disorders: a 5-year outcome study from 16 state physician health programs. Anesth Analg 2009;109: 891–6.

[52] Pelton C, Ikeda RM. The California physician diversion programs experience with recovering anesthesiologists. J Psychoactive Drugs 1991;23:427–31.

[53] Paris RT, Canavan DI. Physician substance abuse impairment: anesthesiologists vs. other specialties. J Addict Dis 1999;18:1–7.

[54] Merk EJ, Baumgarten RK, Kingsley CP, et al. Success of re-entry into anesthesiology training programs by residents with a history of substance abuse. JAMA 1990;263:3060–2.

[55] Bryson EO, Levine A. One approach to return to residency for anesthesia residents recovering from opioid addiction. J Clin Anesth 2008;20:397–400.

[56] Berge KH, Seppala MD, Lanier WL. The anesthesiology community's approach to opioid and anesthetic-abusing personnel: time to change course. Anesthesiology 2008;109: 762–4.

[57] Oreskovich MR, Caldeiro RM. Anesthesiologists recovering from chemical dependency: can they safely return to the operating room? Mayo Clin Proc 2009;84:576–80.

[58] Hedberg EG. Anesthesiologists: addicted to the drugs they administer. ASA Newsl 2001;65:14–6.

[59] Domino KB, Horbein TF, Polissar NL, et al. Risk factors for relapse in health care professionals with substance abuse disorders. JAMA 2005;293:1453–60.

[60] Lutsky I, Abram SE, Jacobsen GR, et al. Substance abuse by anesthesiology residents. Acad Med 1991;66:164–6.

[61] Klein RL, Stevens WC, Kingston HG. Controlled substance dispensing and accountability in United States anesthesiology residency programs. Anesthesiology 1992;77:806–11.

[62] Moleski RJ, Easley S, Barash PG, et al. Control and accountability of controlled substance administration in the operating room. Anesth Analg 1985;64:989–95.

[63] Beljan JR, Bohigian GM, Estes EH, et al. Issues in employee drug testing. JAMA 1987;258: 2089–96.

[64] Orenlicher D. Drug testing of physicians (editorial). JAMA 1990;264:1039–40.

[65] Zwerling C. Current practice and experience in drug and alcohol testing in the workplace. Bull Narc 1999;45:155–96.

[66] Pent MA. Financial viability of screening of drugs of abuse. Clin Chem 1995;41:805–8.

[67] Scott M. Legal aspects of drug testing. ASA Newsl 2005;69:25–8.

[68] Clark HW. The role of physicians as medical review officers in workplace drug testing programs. West J Med 1990;152:514–24.

[69] Fitzsimons MG, Baker KH, Lowenstein E, et al. Random drug testing to reduce the incidence of addition in anesthesia residency: preliminary results from one program. Anesth Analg 2008;107:630–5.

[70] Liang BA. To tell the truth: potential liability for concealing physician impairment. J Clin Anesth 2007;19:638–41.

[71] Liang BA. Responsibility for anesthesiologist suicide relating to drug abuse. J Clin Anesth 2009;21:135–6.

Advances in Anesthesia 29 (2011) 129–148

ADVANCES IN ANESTHESIA

Anesthesia for Intrauterine Fetal Therapy and Ex Utero Intrapartum Therapy

Kha M. Tran, MD

Department of Anesthesia, Fetal Anesthesia Team, Children's Hospital of Philadelphia, University of Pennsylvania School of Medicine, 9th Floor, 34th Street and Civic Center Boulevard, Philadelphia, PA 19104, USA

The concept of treating the fetus as a patient began as early as the 1960s when A.W. Liley, an obstetrician from New Zealand, discovered that he could withdraw ascitic fluid from fetuses suffering heart failure due to red cell alloimmunization. Intraperitoneal transfusion of red blood cells had been previously described in neonates [1]. With this knowledge, Liley was able to medically treat a fetus suffering from hydrops fetalis due to red cell alloimmunization with an intraperitoneal red blood cell transfusion [2].

In the 1980s Michael Harrison, working at the University of California, San Francisco, took the idea of fetal therapy from medical management with transfusions one step further to surgical management [3]. A fetus suffering from bladder outlet obstruction was treated with surgical decompression of his bladder [4].

Advances in diagnostic imaging, such as obstetric ultrasonography and fetal magnetic resonance imaging (MRI), have allowed physicians to diagnose disease in the fetus as it develops in utero. The natural histories of these diseases are being elucidated, and in some cases they are amenable to in utero therapy that can change the progression of disease and prevent fetal demise [5]. In other cases, the fetal disease may not be lethal in utero, but will lead to long-term disability, morbidity and, possibly, mortality. Fetal therapy may change the course of the disease to allow for improved quality of life, with less morbidity and mortality [6]. Finally, some disease processes may not threaten the life of the fetus in utero, but will not allow it to make a successful transition from intrauterine to extrauterine life. Fetal therapy can make that transition possible [7,8].

This work is supported with internal departmental funding.
The author has nothing to disclose.

E-mail address: trank@email.chop.edu

0737-6146/11/$ – see front matter
doi:10.1016/j.aan.2011.07.005

Conducting any anesthetic requires an understanding of the pathophysiology of the disease necessitating surgery, the details of the surgical procedure, and the patient's own physiology. The same principles apply when formulating an anesthetic plan for fetal interventions. Fetal surgical cases are still quite rare when compared with the numbers of other surgical cases being performed, and fetal surgical cases often involve intense collaboration between many subspecialties whose effective communication with each other is essential.

RATIONALE FOR FETAL THERAPY

Three broad classes of disease or disease process may be amenable to therapy. In the first case, the life of fetus is at risk as it develops in utero. Progression of the disease will result in fetal demise. Some examples of these diseases include twin-twin transfusion syndrome [9] or a rapidly growing lung tumor [10,11]. Hydrops fetalis is an end point that may signal the need for fetal intervention. It can be thought of as "fetal heart failure," and is manifested by soft-tissue edema or fluid collections in serous cavities [12]. These collections may include pericardial effusions, pleural effusions, ascites, skin edema, or excessive amniotic fluid (polyhydramnios) [13–15]. Hydrops fetalis can be divided into immune and nonimmune causes. The classic reason for developing immune hydrops is from red cell alloimmunization due to Rh incompatibility. Nonimmune hydrops, which may in some cases require surgical intervention, may be due to cardiac or vascular compression and mass effect from tumors in the thorax [16]; high-output heart failure from rapidly growing sacrococcygeal teratomas [17]; or twin-twin transfusion or reversed arterial perfusion sequence [18].

Second, some diseases, if untreated, will result in disability after birth, and treating the disease earlier in gestation may allow for better growth and development, and less subsequent disability. The primary example of this is fetal closure of myelomeningocele [6]. Treatment of evolving hypoplastic left heart syndrome with balloon dilation of aortic valve stenosis may allow the development of two ventricles [19].

Lastly, some diseases will not allow for successful transition to extrauterine life, and fetal therapy immediately before birth will facilitate neonatal resuscitation. Airway obstruction from tumor or atresia is a typical example of such a disease process. As a fetus, a large airway tumor will not interfere with respiration, as the organ of ventilation is the placenta, but obstruction of the airway may impede breathing of the neonate [8,20]. Securing the airway before clamping the umbilical cord at delivery is a life-saving intervention. Large lung tumors causing mediastinal shift may also impede the neonatal resuscitation and the transition from fetus to neonate [21]. Resection of the tumors will relieve the mediastinal shift and cardiac compression to facilitate neonatal resuscitation.

Maternal mirror syndrome

In some cases of fetal disease, it is not only the life of the fetus at risk but also that of the mother. Some mothers with a fetus suffering from hydrops fetalis may actually develop a constellation of symptoms "mirroring" that of the fetus [22]. The mother may develop hypertension, proteinuria, and life-threatening pulmonary edema. This syndrome has some similarities with preeclampsia. However, hemodilution is more likely with mirror syndrome, and hemoconcentration is more likely to occur with preeclampsia [23]. Treating the cause of the hydrops will treat the maternal mirror syndrome [24].

SPECIFIC DISEASES AND TREATMENTS

Only a handful of diseases are currently amenable to fetal therapy, but the diseases span a wide range of organ systems, ranging from neurologic to cardiovascular to genitourinary. These diseases deserve individual mention to inform the decision making in medical and surgical treatment as well as planning for anesthetic management.

Multiple gestations

Complications of multiple gestations requiring fetal intervention are more common than for any other fetal diseases [18]. Multiple gestations occur in 1 of 90 pregnancies. Twins can be classified as monozygotic or dizygotic. Monozygotic twins are at higher risk for developing complications compared with dizygotic twins. All monozygotic twins can be considered to be "conjoined" at some level, from genetic to physical. After fertilization, monozygotic twinning occurs if the cell mass divides, and it is the timing of the division of the cell mass that determines the degree of conjoinedness. If the zygote divides early enough, two cell masses will implant in the uterus, and the twins will each develop with a separate placenta, chorion, and amnion (dichorionic, diamniotic twins). These twins are "conjoined" at the level of their genes. If the cell mass splits between 3 and 9 days after conception, the twins can share some placental vessels and the chorion (monochorionic, diamniotic twins). These twins are conjoined at the level of their placental vessels and are thus referred to as chorioangiopagus. If the cell mass splits 9 to 13 days after conception, the twins will share both chorion and amnion (monochorionic, monoamniotic twins). Because these twins share the same amniotic space, they are at greater risk for umbilical cord accidents. One step further, and the twins are physically conjoined not only as fetuses but also after birth. Twinning 13 or more days after fertilization will result in what are typically thought of as conjoined twins, who may be conjoined at the head, thorax, abdomen, or pelvis (craniopagus, thoracopagus, omphalopagus, or ischiopagus).

It is the chorioangiopagus twins that may suffer from diseases amenable to fetal intervention. The placental vessels that are shared between the twins allow for blood flow between the twins, and this blood flow may be unbalanced such that there is a net flow of blood from one twin (the donor) to the other (the recipient). The donor twin may develop hypovolemia and oligohydramnios, and is at risk for growth restriction. The recipient is at risk for hypervolemia, polyhydramnios, and congestive heart failure. Both twins are at risk for death and neurologic complications, such as periventricular leukomalacia. This disease process is called twin-twin transfusion syndrome (TTTS). Historically, treatment of TTTS consists of serial amnioreductions in the twin that suffers from polyhydramnios to relieve increased intrauterine pressure and hopefully allow increased fetal perfusion, and also hopefully to lower the incidence of preterm labor [9]. This approach represents symptomatic therapy, and newer approaches are targeting the pathophysiology of this disease by ablating the placental vessels that allow the unbalanced blood flow. This ablation of placental vessels, in the proper patient population and with skilled procedural-ists, seems to be more effective at preventing death, preterm labor, and neuro-logic complications [25,26].

In some cases one of the twins does not develop a heart or a brain, and acts as a "parasite." The normal twin must supply cardiac output both for itself and also for the acardiac cell mass via the placental vessels that are connected. This extra cardiac workload places the normal twin at risk for high-output cardiac failure. In these cases, a technically simpler procedure is performed in which the umbilical cord of the acardiac cell mass is occluded, by either bipolar cautery or radiofrequency ablation [27,28].

These procedures are minimally invasive, typically using fetoscopes ranging in size from 1 to 3.8 mm in diameter [29]. Ultrasound and fetoscopes are used alone or in conjunction to guide the bipolar cautery, radiofrequency probes, or fiberoptic laser cables to their targets.

Airway

Extrinsic compression of the airway may result from tumors such as teratomas or lymphangiomas, whereas intrinsic airway obstruction results from airway agenesis or atresia, cysts, or webs [20,30]. Because not all tumors will cause life-threatening airway obstruction, the fetal imaging studies must be inter-preted carefully, and delivery plans should be made in a multidisciplinary manner, involving nurses, surgeons, anesthesiologists, neonatologists, and the family. If the fetus is deemed to be at significant risk for severe obstruction, the airway must be secured before birth during ex utero intrapartum therapy (EXIT procedure). The EXIT procedure occurs in late gestation and involves a maternal laparotomy, hysterotomy, and fetal airway control before the umbil-ical cord is cut. By continuing to use the placenta as the organ of respiration, the airway can be evaluated and secured in a controlled fashion over the course of an hour or more. The extra time allows for direct laryngoscopy, rigid bron-choscopy, oral intubation, tracheostomy, tumor debulking, and even neck dissection with retrograde wire intubation [7,8,31]. It is only after the airway is secured that the child is delivered to a team of neonatologists for completion of the newborn resuscitation.

The range of causes of intrinsic airway obstruction has been collectively called congenital high airway obstruction syndrome [30]. Laryngeal cysts and webs, or atresia of parts of the airway, also require close study and multi-disciplinary delivery planning [32]. An EXIT procedure may be required before delivery of the child. Intrinsic airway obstruction poses a unique threat to the life of the fetus, not just at the time of delivery but also during development. In cases of total fetal airway obstruction, the fluid produced by the developing lungs has no egress. The lungs may become distended with fluid, and may compress the heart and great vessels. This compression can be conceptualized as a "tension hydrothorax," with subsequent fetal heart failure and death [30]. Treatment of this severe form of airway obstruction can include laser decompression of the fetal trachea to allow egress of lung fluid [33].

Lung

Lung tumors such as bronchopulmonary sequestration (BPS) and congenital cystic adenomatoid malformation (CCAM) have variable natural histories, and large lesions may require fetal therapy at various stages of gestation [11]. CCAM and BPS cause problems in utero by exerting mass effect on the heart and great vessels. Severe compression will result in mediastinal shift, hydrops fetalis, and fetal demise. Tumors may have components that are macrocystic, microcystic, or both. Some tumors remain small, some grow aggressively, and some grow and regress. Symptomatic compression may occur in early, middle, or late gestation [34].

Given the variable natural history, these lesions must be followed closely, at times requiring twice-weekly fetal ultrasonography and possibly serial fetal echocardiography. The management of prenatally diagnosed CCAM is illustrative of the dynamic nature of fetal therapy. Small lesions that do not grow aggressively do not require fetal intervention, and an elective thoracotomy and lobectomy can be scheduled several months after delivery. Large lesions causing hydrops should be treated. A large macrocystic lesion may be treated minimally invasively with ultrasound-guided needle aspiration. If fluid reaccumulates in the cyst, it may need to be treated with chronic drainage. A thoracoamniotic shunt, which will allow chronic drainage, can be placed with ultrasound guidance [34]. Microcystic lesions are not amenable to drainage. If a large CCAM with microcystic components is causing hydrops in the middle of gestation with immature lungs, primary resection is the treatment of choice. This approach involves a maternal laparotomy and hysterotomy. The fetus is partially exposed, and a thoracotomy is performed for fetal pulmonary lobectomy. A major difference in this surgery when compared with an EXIT procedure is that the fetus is then replaced in the uterus for further growth and development. If the microcystic tumor does not become symptomatic until later in gestation and the lungs are mature, an EXIT procedure is the treatment option of choice. Some of these large lung tumors cause mediastinal shift, compress the heart and great vessels, and impede ventilation after the child is born. In select cases, the child is better served by thoracotomy and removal of the tumor immediately before birth during an EXIT procedure [21].

Previous attempts at fetal therapy for congenital diaphragmatic hernia have not been shown to be better than optimal postnatal therapy [35]. Trials with even more minimally invasive therapy for diaphragmatic hernia are being conducted in Europe and will be beginning in the United States [36].

Cardiac

The list of cardiac diseases that are actually or theoretically amenable to fetal cardiac intervention is growing. The majority of the human experience has been with aortic valvuloplasty, pulmonary valvuloplasty, and atrial septoplasty [19]. It has been hypothesized that cardiac valvular disease in the fetus may have an impact on the proper development of the cardiac chambers. Specifically, some cases of fetal aortic stenosis impeding flow out of the developing left ventricle may evolve into hypoplastic left heart syndrome [37,38]. Treating the aortic stenosis in the middle of gestation may allow cardiac growth and development of a two-ventricle heart. The same logic applies to treating pulmonary atresia with an intact ventricular septum, as it may evolve into hypoplastic right heart syndrome. Other cardiac disease, such as hypoplastic left heart with an intact or highly restrictive atrial septum, may require intervention to allow decompression of the left atrium [39].

The surgical approach to fetal cardiac intervention has evolved. Early cases included a laparotomy without hysterotomy, and minimally invasive access to the fetal heart with catheters and needles introduced through the uterus, directly into the cardiac chambers via the fetal chest wall. As more experience is accumulating, many fetal cardiac interventions are now completed with entirely minimally invasive techniques, involving needles and catheters inserted percutaneously through the maternal abdomen [40].

Neurologic

This area of fetal therapy has experienced failure in the past, but has met with recent success. Ventriculoamniotic shunting for obstructive hydrocephalus in a fetus is a logical development of the widely accepted use of ventriculoperitoneal shunting for obstructive hydrocephalus, but the outcomes of these fetal procedures have not been successful [41]. As a confounding factor, many fetuses presenting with obstructive hydrocephalus have a host of other comorbidities that can affect the fetal outcome. On the other hand, midgestation repair of myelomeningocele has recently been shown to be an effective therapy that decreases the need for ventriculoperitoneal shunting and improves neurologic motor function [6]. The rationale for treating myelomeningocele in utero is based on protection of the spinal cord from damage by exposure to amniotic fluid [42–44]. This procedure is an open fetal surgical procedure performed around 24 weeks gestation and involves maternal laparotomy, hysterotomy, exposure of the fetal myelomeningocele, and closure of the defect. This closure can be primary, but large defects may require allograft. The fetus is then replaced in the uterus and delivered via cesarean section closer to term.

Genitourinary

Lower urinary tract obstruction can have wide-ranging implications in a fetus, and include dilated bladder, hydroureter, hydronephrosis, and eventual renal parenchymal damage [45]. Urinary tract obstruction contributes to oligohydramnios or even anhydramnios, which can cause skeletal abnormalities and pulmonary hypoplasia. Decompression of the urinary tract is the goal of therapy in these cases, and it can usually be accomplished minimally invasively with serial aspirations or vesicoamniotic shunting. Open fetal surgical approaches have been described [46]. Some of the impediments to progress in this field are attributable to very challenging patient selection criteria. The fetus must be "sick enough" to warrant an intervention, but the disease must not have progressed so far that the renal or other damage is irreversible. Workup involves fetal imaging and testing of fetal urinary electrolytes.

Sacrococcygeal teratoma

Rapidly growing sacrococcygeal teratomas place the fetus at risk of death from high-output heart failure secondary to a "steal" phenomenon, in which the tumor causes increased work for the fetal heart [47]. In addition to the steal phenomenon, the tumor may rupture in utero and cause fetal anemia [17]. Cystic tumors are not typically as problematic as solid tumors. If a fetus is going into heart failure in the middle of gestation, treatment is warranted, but the tumor size, shape, and location must be favorable. Minimally invasive approaches have not as yet been successful [48], but open debulking of these tumors has been performed [49]. In late gestation, another option is a planned cesarean delivery with immediate access to an adjacent operating room for immediate resection to avoid the risk of tumor rupture, although in cases of massive tumors even this approach may not succeed [50].

PHYSIOLOGIC CONSIDERATIONS FOR ANESTHETIC MANAGEMENT

As with all anesthetics, understanding the physiology of the patient, the requirements of the surgical procedure, and the physiologic effects of administered drugs is crucial. A unique consideration in fetal therapy is that the surgery involves two patients. Both of these patients, a parturient and a fetus, are at higher than usual anesthetic risk, and they must be cared for simultaneously. Some models for anesthetic care involve both an obstetric and pediatric anesthesia team to care for the mother and fetus, respectively. Some models involve only one anesthesia team caring simultaneously for the mother and fetus. These types of management decisions can be made on an individual basis, or may be dependent on the culture and infrastructure of the particular institution where the fetal procedure is being performed.

Changes during pregnancy

The physiologic changes during pregnancy should be familiar to the majority of anesthesiologists. The brief treatment of this subject does not diminish the importance of these changes in determining the anesthetic management, but reflects the wide availability of obstetric anesthetic resources.

Although many anesthetic dosing requirements are decreased during pregnancy [51] this does not typically change anesthetic management, because high-dose volatile anesthetic agents are commonly used in open fetal surgery [52], and relatively high doses of sedatives can be given to mothers for fetal sedation [53,54]. As pregnancy increases the risk of pulmonary aspiration of gastric contents [55], aspiration prophylaxis for women undergoing maternal-fetal surgery should be routine. Not all cases require general endotracheal anesthesia, but the anesthesia team should be prepared for rapid sequence induction and intubation. Capillary engorgement of the airway mucosa may contribute to more difficult airway management [56–58]. Functional residual capacity is decreased [59], oxygen consumption is increased, and pregnant patients are more prone to rapid arterial oxygen desaturation. The compensated respiratory alkalosis of pregnancy should be kept in mind when managing ventilation. Cardiac output increases [60], systemic vascular resistance decreases, and both plasma and red blood cell volume increase. Aortocaval compression from the gravid uterus may predispose patients to supine hypotension. Pregnancy induces a state of increased, compensated intravascular coagulation. Patients are at increased risk for venous thrombosis.

Uteroplacental physiology

The placenta acts as the interface between the mother and fetus for the transport of drugs, oxygen, nutrients, and waste products. Maternal spiral arteries deposit oxygen-rich blood into the intervillus space. Deoxygenated fetal blood travels to the placenta via the umbilical arteries, which branch into arterioles and capillaries and enter the placenta where oxygen is bound and waste products are deposited, in much the same way that deoxygenated blood travels to the lungs from via the pulmonary arteries. Oxygenated blood then travels back to the fetus via the umbilical vein.

To ensure adequate perfusion of the fetus, adequate blood flow must be maintained through the uterus, placenta, and umbilical cord. A breakdown in any part of this chain can put the fetus at risk. Uterine blood flow is proportional to the difference between uterine arterial pressure and venous pressure, and uterine blood flow is inversely proportional to uterine vascular resistance. Maternal hypotension will decrease arterial pressure, increased uterine muscle tone will increase uterine vascular resistance, and aortocaval compression will both decrease arterial pressure and increase venous pressure. Maternal hypercapnea may increase uterine blood flow [61–63]. Thus, many factors have a variable effect on uterine blood flow, and their use and effects must be balanced in maternal-fetal surgery. Volatile anesthetics will certainly decrease uterine tone and vascular resistance, but systemic blood pressure will also be decreased [64]. Vasopressors may increase systemic blood pressure, but simultaneously increase vascular resistance. Vasodilators may decrease uterine vascular resistance but also decrease systemic blood pressure. Neuraxial anesthetics may allow increased uterine blood flow, but only as long as systemic blood pressure is maintained [65]. In sum, management decisions, hemodynamic changes, and manipulations must allow for adequate fetal perfusion, as can be monitored by fetal heart rate, pulse oximetry, echocardiography, and blood gas analysis.

The uteroplacental interface must remain intact. Placental abruption is a risk if the uterine tone is too high, or if amniotic fluid volume is lost too rapidly after hysterotomy is made. The placenta may implant anywhere on the inner surface of the uterus, and the location of the placenta will have great impact on the location of any planned access to the fetus, whether by hysterotomy or minimally invasive technique. Physical pressure from surgeons or their instruments may decrease blood flow and fetal perfusion.

The physiology of the umbilical cord itself is not complex, but it must remain patent. Kinking or compression of the umbilical cord will negate any of the upstream efforts made by the anesthesia team toward maximizing fetal perfusion. Kinking or compression may be subclinical or acute, and is commonly caused by surgical instruments used to expose the fetus, surgeons' hands as they are positioning the fetus, or the fetus itself if amniotic fluid volume is rapidly lost.

Drug transport across the placenta is a concern during pregnancy. In most cases, the concern involves avoiding inappropriate fetal drug exposure [66]. In the case of fetal surgery, the anesthesiologist is often trying to deliver medications to the fetus and, while several routes of administration are possible, maternal intravenous administration is the most common and technically simple. Smaller, lipophilic drugs cross the placenta more readily than larger, polarized drugs.

Fetal physiology

Rigorous study of human fetal physiology is difficult for a variety of practical and ethical reasons. As such, our understanding of the impact of anesthetic management on fetal physiology comes from a combination of direct human study, extension of human preterm neonatal data, and animal studies.

Neurologic

The fetal neurologic system is immature. Two important issues arise from this fact, and many hard questions remain to be answered. The first is potential neurotoxicity of anesthetic agents on the developing brain [67] and the second is fetal pain perception [68,69]. Neurotoxicity in the developing brain is an important topic for study in the whole discipline of pediatric anesthesia, and the implications of studies in this field will likely affect the field of fetal anesthesia, as the fetal brain is probably even more sensitive to potentially damaging effects of anesthetic agents. Newborn rats, when exposed to agents such as isoflurane, midazolam, and nitrous oxide for prolonged periods of time, have shown evidence of increased apoptosis of neural cells, and these rats have also not performed as well in tests of neurologic function [70]. Great caution must be exercised in the extrapolation of studies such as this, for several reasons. These studies are on animals, the rats are not monitored as carefully as a human is during a surgical procedure, and the relative length of exposure in such studies is much greater than a human undergoing surgery. Nevertheless, the concern about doing harm to humans is a real one. Some solace flows from the facts that there are few other options for agents to provide anesthesia, and any newer options for drugs are likely to have their potential effects even less well characterized than the current armamentarium. Much work remains to be done in this field [71].

Fetal pain perception is a controversial topic. The subjective component of pain makes studies even in adult humans challenging. The fact of neonatal pain is no longer seen as controversial, but it has taken years of study to come to this point [72]. It will take much more work to be able to make conclusive statements about fetal pain. Invasive fetal procedures can be done as early as 18 weeks, and can be done quite close to term in the case of EXIT procedures. Although the neural structures required for processing pain do not form until approximately 26 weeks' gestation [73], seeing a premature baby born at 25 weeks' gestation withdraw to heel sticks in the neonatal intensive care unit can certainly color the practitioner's opinion. These observations, however, cannot yet be confidently translated into understanding the experience of fetal pain and its treatment.

Whereas concepts of fetal pain are controversial, the concept of a fetal stress response is not. When a human fetus is subjected to an invasive procedure such as an intrahepatic blood transfusion, a needle is passed though the fetal abdominal wall into hepatic vessels. Measured levels of "stress hormones," such as cortisol and endorphins, are increased [74]. Cardiovascular changes also occur, such as an increase in the pulsatility index of the fetal middle cerebral artery, commonly interpreted as a hemodynamic response to fetal stress. Administration of fentanyl to fetuses in these circumstances will attenuate or ablate these measurements of stress response [74]. The ill effects of a fetal stress response can only be extrapolated from the ill effects of a neonatal stress response.

Cardiac physiology

No discussion of fetal cardiac physiology would be complete without a description of the fetal circulation. Oxygenated blood leaves the placenta and travels to the fetus via the umbilical vein. Some of the oxygenated blood bypasses the liver as it travels to the heart via the ductus venosus. As the blood enters the heart, most is shunted from the right atrium across the foramen ovale into the left atrium, and some goes to the right ventricle. There is relatively less flow of blood from the right ventricle to the lungs because blood from the right ventricle is preferentially shunted from the pulmonary artery across the ductus arteriosus to the aorta. Blood leaving the left atrium enters the left ventricle and exits the heart via the aorta. The blood supplying the head has greater oxygen saturation than blood supplying the lower body. Deoxygenated blood returns to the heart via the superior and inferior vena cavae.

The heart muscle itself is less contractile and less organized than that of more mature myocardium. It is also less able to respond to increases in preload with increases in contractility [75]. Blood in a normal adult human flows in series. The fetus is differentiated by blood that flows in parallel because of the 3 shunts that are present: the ductus venosus, the foramen ovale, and the ductus arteriosus. Because the blood flows in parallel, the cardiac output of the fetal heart must be described by the combined cardiac output (CCO) of both ventricles.

The normal range of the CCO in a fetus is approximately 425 to 550 mL/kg/min [76]. Fetal echocardiography is done frequently in fetuses at risk for high-output heart failure, and the CCO can reach values as high as 900 mL/kg/min or more.

Pulmonary physiology
Ventilation is not a consideration in the pulmonary physiology of the fetus, as pulmonary blood flow is minimal and no gas exchange occurs in the fetal lungs. The aspect of pulmonary physiology that most affects the neonate is the production of lung fluid. This fluid is made by the lungs, and in most cases exits the lungs via the trachea to contribute to amniotic fluid volume. When the egress of this fluid is interrupted, pathologic states can develop that will place the fetus at risk for heart failure, as the lungs will become distended and interfere with cardiac function [30].

Hematologic considerations
The small blood volume in a fetus leaves little margin for blood loss during invasive procedures. In early gestation (16–22 weeks) the fetus and placenta combined have a blood volume ranging from 120 to 160 mL/kg [77,78]. A fetus at 16 weeks' gestation weighs about 100 g. At 31 weeks, a fetus has a blood volume of about 90 mL/kg. A fetus at 31 weeks weighs approximately 500 g. Although the actual blood type of the fetus cannot be determined without performing a fetal type and screen, maternal antibodies to red blood cell antigens can cross the placenta. The risk of obtaining fetal blood for typing outweighs the benefit, as type O-negative blood can be given, and the volumes that would be given, usually less than a quarter of a unit of packed red blood cells, would not constitute a large drain on the resources of a blood bank. Any blood given to the fetus, however, should be cross-matched against a maternal blood sample to test for antibodies. Thus, the fetus receives O-negative, cross-matched blood. The coagulation system continues to mature well into the neonatal period. Mean prothrombin time for a fetus between 24 and 29 weeks is 32.2 seconds. Mean activated partial thromboplastin time at this gestational age is 154.0 seconds [79].

Thermoregulation
Temperature control during minimally invasive cases is not typically a management challenge, but it is important during open fetal cases. The skin barrier of a fetus is not yet developed, shivering and nonshivering thermogenesis responses are absent in utero [80], and evaporative losses will be increased as the fetus is undergoing surgical procedures while in a bath of amniotic fluid. As much of the fetus as possible is kept submerged in the amniotic fluid to prevent such heat loss.

ANESTHETIC PLANS
With the foundations laid by understanding the fetal/maternal physiology and the basics of the fetal pathophysiology, the next step is communication with all team members to come up with a sound anesthetic plan. These procedures can

be resource-intensive with respect to equipment, medications, space and, most importantly, people. The multidisciplinary nature of fetal therapy cannot be over-emphasized, as the team members involved in the procedure may include obstetric anesthesiologists, pediatric anesthesiologists, pediatric general surgeons, pediatric otolaryngologists, operating room nurses, obstetricians, perinatologists, obstetric nurses, neonatologists, neonatal nurses, invasive and noninvasive cardiologists, cardiac catheterization laboratory nurses, perfusionists and, most importantly, a highly motivated family with strong support systems in place. Roles of the team members should be clearly defined. Primary plans and contingency plans must be in place in case the fetus does not tolerate the procedure. Common resources such as blood or medications need to be easily accessible by all. Team members all should have an understanding of the roles and capabilities of the other members.

Preoperative preparation

These cases are complex, and both the fetus and mother are at increased anesthetic risk. While the goal is the help the fetus, the mother must also undergo a surgical procedure and, in most cases, does not stand to reap any direct benefits (an exception is the case of maternal mirror syndrome, where treating the fetus will also improve the health of the mother). Mothers must be seen preoperatively for counseling and for anesthetic risk stratification. These procedures should be undertaken only very cautiously if the mother has any serious comorbidities. A standard anesthetic history and physical should be supplemented with a focused airway and spine examination, in addition to specific questions about severity of gastroesophageal reflux, supine hypotension, and a history of anesthetic complications. The most recent estimated fetal weight should be noted if medications are to be given directly to the fetus, and the location of the placenta should be noted, as this will affect patient positioning and the surgical approach in many cases. All fetal studies should be reviewed, including ultrasonography, MRI, and echocardiography. A maternal type and screen is done for minimally invasive cases, and cross-matching 2 to 4 units of packed red blood cells for the mother and a small aliquot of blood for the fetus is helpful in open fetal cases if fetal bleeding is expected. Further laboratory, imaging, or diagnostic studies should be dictated by the clinical situation of each patient.

All patients should receive aspiration prophylaxis. As the goal in many fetal cases is to have a "sedated" or anesthetized fetus and the level of preoperative anxiety in these cases is often quite high, judicious dosing of midazolam in the preoperative period is often helpful. In many cases the mother will also receive oral or rectal indomethacin preoperatively to aid with tocolysis.

Team meetings should be held before fetal surgical procedures to go over details with the team and the family. Any outstanding issues can be addressed at these meetings.

Minimally invasive procedures

These procedures, while typically not as resource-intensive as open fetal cases, still require close communication because there is a wide range of therapeutic possibilities and outcomes. As these cases are so variable, all the possibilities cannot often be discussed in detail. Some examples are given here, illustrating the factors considered when developing the anesthetic plan. Standard monitoring is used for the mother, and fetal monitoring consists of real time ultrasound determination of the fetal heart rate.

Laser ablation of placental vessels
In cases of laser ablation of placental vessels for TTTS, local anesthesia is used for the maternal abdomen, the instruments are relatively small, and having fetuses that are not vigorously moving makes the procedure technically easier for the surgeon. Complete paralysis is typically not needed in these cases. Given these needs, administration of medications to the mother for passage to the fetus is a common technique. Traditionally a combination of morphine and diazepam has been used. Although pregnant women are more sensitive to anesthetic agents, 10 to 20 mg each of morphine and diazepam is not unusual. Quicker-acting medications, such as propofol, fentanyl, midazolam, and remifentanil, are also used. The doses should be carefully titrated, and the risk of aspiration or hypoventilation should be considered in these cases. The author prefers a bolus of 2 to 3 mg of midazolam after the patient has lay down on the bed. Initiating an infusion of remifentanil at 0.1 μg/kg/min without a bolus typically provides a satisfactory plane of anesthesia, with the mother still able to converse and help position themselves if the access to the placental vessels is challenging.

Fetal cardiac interventions
At the other end of the spectrum of minimally invasive fetal cases is a fetal atrial septostomy. Whereas some patient movement can be tolerated for correction of twin-twin transfusion, no movement can be tolerated during fetal cardiac catheterization. These cases were formerly performed on an intact uterus after surgeons performed a laparotomy. If a laparotomy were being planned, a high lumbar or low thoracic epidural would provide postoperative analgesia. Techniques and skills have improved, and most of these procedures can now be performed completely percutaneously [81]. Because maternal movement cannot be tolerated, general endotracheal anesthesia is usually chosen. The fetus is often given an injection of fentanyl and vecuronium. Because the needles are introduced into the fetal myocardium fetal arrhythmias are common, and the team should have rescue doses of atropine and epinephrine available.

Open midgestation procedures
The procedure
These procedures are much more labor-intensive and resource-intensive. However, there is not as broad a range of therapeutic options in these cases, so the anesthetic can be more standardized. The majority of these cases will be for elective closure of a fetal myelomeningocele or for semiurgent resection of tumors causing hydrops. After maternal laparotomy, sterile intraoperative ultrasonography is used to map the edges of the placenta so that the

hysterotomy can be made to avoid it. If the placenta is implanted on the anterior surface of the uterus, this will necessitate complete exteriorization of the uterus, with a uterine incision on the posterior aspect of the uterus. Special stapling devices are deployed to prevent bleeding from the edges of the uterus. Amniotic fluid will invariably leak out of the hysterotomy, and this is replaced with warmed lactated Ringer solution administered via a rapid infusing system into a red rubber catheter that is placed into the uterine cavity. Fetal monitoring depends on the case, and may range from as minimal as intermittent fetal heart rates obtained by ultrasound, to complete monitoring with fetal pulse oximetry and sterile intraoperative echocardiography. Normal fetal oxygen saturations are 40% to 70%. In some cases the fetus will receive a peripheral intravenous catheter. In most cases the fetus will also receive an intramuscular injection of medications, typically including fentanyl (20 μg/kg), atropine (20 μg/kg), and vecuronium (0.2 mg/kg). The fetal procedure is completed, the fetal skin is closed, any fetal catheters or monitors are removed, and the fetus is replaced in the uterus. The mother's abdomen is then closed.

The anesthetic

After initial intravenous access is obtained, a high lumbar or low thoracic epidural is placed for postoperative analgesia. A test dose is given, but the epidural is not yet bolused with local anesthetic. After aspiration prophylaxis, the mother is placed supine with left uterine displacement and standard monitors. After preoxygenation/denitrogenation she is intubated after rapid sequence induction of general anesthesia. Large-bore intravenous access is placed. Although these cases are generally not bloody because of the special uterine staples, when hemorrhage happens it happens quickly, as the gravid uterus has almost 1000 mL/min of blood flow [82] and the effects of volatile anesthetics will increase uterine blood loss [83]. Invasive arterial blood pressure monitoring is necessary in these cases because small changes in maternal blood pressure can have a dramatic physiologic effect on the fetus. The blood pressure must be maintained very close to baseline to allow adequate fetoplacental perfusion. Complicating the management of the maternal blood pressure are the competing goals of uterine relaxation and avoidance of pulmonary edema.

Intense uterine relaxation is a hallmark of open fetal cases. The goal is to minimize uterine vascular resistance and allow for fetal perfusion as long as blood pressure is maintained. High uterine tone will also cause rapid loss of amniotic fluid as the hysterotomy is made, and this rapid loss of fluid can increase the risk of umbilical cord compression or even placental abruption. A relaxed uterus will also make surgical access and positioning easier. Preoperative indomethacin is given to aid with intraoperative uterine relaxation. The medications commonly used to achieve uterine relaxation intraoperatively include high-dose volatile anesthetic agents and nitroglycerin. The concentrations of volatile anesthetic are typically twice the normal minimum alveolar concentration. Any volatile agent can be used, but desflurane, with its low blood/gas partition coefficient, affords the advantage of rapid offset in the case of maternal bleeding. Nitroglycerin can be given as either an intermittent bolus or an infusion [84]. After the fetal procedure is complete and the uterus is being closed, the volatile anesthetic is weaned at the same time a magnesium sulfate bolus is administered.

Women undergoing fetal surgery appear to be at greater risk for pulmonary edema [85], which may be due to the heavy postoperative tocolytic regimens or unknown factors that are released from the uterus during manipulation and incision. Given this risk of pulmonary edema, the typical fluid management for an open midgestation case is very restrictive. An average-sized patient receives about 500mL crystalloid for the whole case. Hypotension is to be expected when a mother is receiving high-dose volatile anesthetic, with or without nitroglycerin, and can only get 500mL of crystalloid. Assuming other causes of hypotension have been excluded or treated, the drug-induced hypotension can be treated with standard vasopressors, phenylephrine and ephedrine. Infusions of phenylephrine, in particular, help maintain smooth hemodynamics while minimizing extra fluid administration needed to give repeated boluses of vasopressors.

EXIT procedure

The EXIT procedure has many similarities to a midgestation open fetal procedure, with the major difference being that the child is delivered at the end of the procedure. The maternal laparotomy and hysterotomy are performed, and the fetus undergoes whatever procedure is planned during the EXIT to give the fetus a better chance at successfully transitioning to neonatal physiology. These procedures may include a direct laryngoscopy, rigid bronchoscopy, intubation, neck dissection, tracheostomy, pulmonary lobectomy, or even cannulation for extracorporeal membrane oxygenation [21,86,87]. After the procedure is completed the umbilical cord is clamped and cut, and the child is delivered to the neonatal team for resuscitation. In some cases the fetus does not tolerate the procedure, or it cannot be completed for various reasons, such as intraoperative placental abruption. In these cases, the umbilical cord must be quickly clamped and cut and, if possible, the fetus must be taken to a second operating room for completion of the procedure. Because the primary plan is to deliver the child, coordination with the neonatal team is particularly important, and the team must be ready and present either in the mother's operating room, an adjacent operating room, or a specially prepared neonatal resuscitation room. Because the backup plan is to take the neonate emergently for surgery, the adjacent operating room must be prepared with the proper equipment and staffed with another team of nurses, technicians, and anesthesia providers. As the surgical team for the mother typically includes both pediatric surgeons and an obstetrician or perinatologist, the pediatric surgical team can follow the baby while the obstetric surgical team stays with the mother.

In preparation for the fetal surgical procedure, the anesthesia team should have a sterile pulse oximeter probe and cable that can be applied to the fetus in the surgical field. The cables can then be passed over the drapes and attached to a second pulse oximeter module. Normal fetal heart rate is 120 to 160 beats/min, and normal fetal oxygen saturations are 40% to 70% [88]. It may be beneficial for the fetus to receive a peripheral intravenous catheter in many EXIT procedures. If this is planned, the anesthesia team should have an intravenous fluid line set up for connection to sterile tubing on the field. The intravenous crystalloid should be warmed, and it need not contain dextrose, as the fetus receives glucose from the mother while the placenta is intact. During some cases, particularly for pulmonary lobectomy, the fetus is also intubated before the beginning of the thoracotomy. After intubation, the endotracheal tube should be sutured in place but the fetus should not be ventilated. The goal is to have an airway in place for ventilation after the lobectomy or in case the EXIT cannot be completed, requiring that the child be taken to another operating room. If the fetus were to be ventilated before procedure completion, the cascade of events leading from fetal to neonatal physiology begins prematurely, and may adversely affect the success of the EXIT procedure. It is not helpful to begin increasing pulmonary blood flow by ventilation of the fetus before large areas of diseased lung are resected. After completion of the procedure the fetus is ventilated, and chest rise along with an increase in oxygen saturation confirms correct placement of the endotracheal tube.

Medications and blood should also be prepared for the fetus. The fetus will typically receive the same intramuscular injection of fentanyl, vecuronium, and atropine as a fetus undergoing a midgestation procedure. Emergency doses of atropine, epinephrine, and other medications as needed may be drawn up and given in a sterile fashion to the scrub nurses for administration in the field (intramuscular or via an umbilical vein). Medications may also be given intravenously to the fetus if a peripheral venous catheter has been inserted. Intravenous medication infusions for the fetus have not been used in this author's experience, but there may certainly be a role for infusions in selected cases. Blood, as mentioned previously, should be type O-negative and cross-matched against the mother's blood sample. It should be readily available depending on the needs of the case, and is more likely to be given during tumor debulking or pulmonary lobectomy. As a practical matter, a separate pole for the fetal fluids, blood products, and infusions will limit confusion during the procedure, and will also make transition to a separate operating room much smoother, should that be necessary.

FUTURE DIRECTIONS

Fetal surgery is still evolving. The surgical techniques had a solid preclinical foundation with animal models and basic science. The anesthetic techniques in humans are based on the clinical experience with obstetric and neonatal patients, and the integration of this experience with knowledge of fetal physiology and pathophysiology. Much remains to be studied. As experience grows, the incidence of maternal pulmonary edema seems to be decreasing, although it can still be a problem. Optimal anesthetic techniques to relax the uterus while preserving myocardial function remain to be studied. The pharmacokinetics of the anesthetic medicines in a fetus remain to be described, and further work is indicated to delineate the role of anesthetic agents in neurotoxic effects on the immature nervous system and in limiting the fetal stress response to surgical interventions.

References

[1] Scopes JW. Intraperitoneal transfusion of blood in newborn babies. Lancet 1963;1(7289): 1027–8.

[2] Liley AW. Intrauterine transfusion of foetus in haemolytic disease. Br Med J 1963;2(5365): 1107–9.

[3] Harrison MR, Golbus MS, Filly RA. Management of the fetus with a correctable congenital defect. JAMA 1981;246(7):774–7.

[4] Harrison MR, Golbus MS, Filly RA, et al. Fetal surgery for congenital hydronephrosis. N Engl J Med 1982;306(10):591–3.

[5] Harrison MR. Surgically correctable fetal disease. Am J Surg 2000;180(5):335–42.

[6] Adzick NS, Thom EA, Spong CY, et al. A randomized trial of prenatal versus postnatal repair of myelomeningocele. N Engl J Med 2011;364(11):993–1004.

[7] Mychaliska GB, Bealer JF, Graf JL, et al. Operating on placental support: the ex utero intrapartum treatment procedure. J Pediatr Surg 1997;32(2):227–30 [discussion: 230–1].

[8] Tanaka M, Sato S, Naito H, et al. Anaesthetic management of a neonate with prenatally diagnosed cervical tumour and upper airway obstruction. Can J Anaesth 1994;41(3): 236–40.

[9] Hecher K, Diehl W, Zikulnig L, et al. Endoscopic laser coagulation of placental anastomoses in 200 pregnancies with severe mid-trimester twin-to-twin transfusion syndrome. Eur J Obstet Gynecol Reprod Biol 2000;92(1):135–9.

[10] Brown MF, Lewis D, Brouillette RM, et al. Successful prenatal management of hydrops, caused by congenital cystic adenomatoid malformation, using serial aspirations. J Pediatr Surg 1995;30(7):1098–9.

[11] Adzick NS, Flake AW, Crombleholme TM. Management of congenital lung lesions. Semin Pediatr Surg 2003;12(1):10–6.

[12] Holzgreve W, Holzgreve B, Curry CJ. Nonimmune hydrops fetalis: diagnosis and management. Semin Perinatol 1985;9(2):52–67.

[13] Gordon H. The diagnosis of hydrops fetalis. Clin Obstet Gynecol 1971;14(2):548–60.

[14] Bellini C, Hennekam RC, Fulcheri E, et al. Etiology of nonimmune hydrops fetalis: a systematic review. Am J Med Genet 2009;149A(5):844–51.

[15] Shenker L, Reed KL, Anderson CF, et al. Fetal pericardial effusion. Am J Obstet Gynecol 1989;160(6):1505–7 [discussion: 1507–8].

[16] Adzick NS. Management of fetal lung lesions. Clin Perinatol 2003;30(3):481–92.

[17] Flake AW. Fetal sacrococcygeal teratoma. Semin Pediatr Surg 1993;2(2):113–20.

[18] Lewi L, Van Schoubroeck D, Gratacós E, et al. Monochorionic diamniotic twins: complications and management options. Curr Opin Obstet Gynecol 2003;15(2):177–94.

[19] McElhinney DB, Tworetzky W, Lock JE. Current status of fetal cardiac intervention. Circulation 2010;121(10):1256–63.

[20] Bouchard S. The EXIT procedure: experience and outcome in 31 cases. J Pediatr Surg 2002;37(3):418–26.

[21] Hedrick HL, Flake AW, Crombleholme TM, et al. The ex utero intrapartum therapy procedure for high-risk fetal lung lesions. J Pediatr Surg 2005;40(6):1038–43 [discussion: 1044].

[22] Vidaeff AC, Pschirrer ER, Mastrobattista JM, et al. Mirror syndrome. A case report. J Reprod Med 2002;47(9):770–4.

[23] van Selm M, Kanhai HH, Gravenhorst JB. Maternal hydrops syndrome: a review. Obstet Gynecol Surv 1991;46(12):785–8.

[24] Heyborne KD, Chism DM. Reversal of Ballantyne syndrome by selective second-trimester fetal termination. A case report. J Reprod Med 2000;45(4):360–2.

[25] Senat M, Deprest J, Boulvain M, et al. Endoscopic laser surgery versus serial amnioreduction for severe twin-to-twin transfusion syndrome. N Engl J Med 2004;351(2):136–44.

[26] Crombleholme TM, Shera D, Lee H, et al. A prospective, randomized, multicenter trial of amnioreduction vs selective fetoscopic laser photocoagulation for the treatment of severe twin-twin transfusion syndrome. Am J Obstet Gynecol 2007;197(4):396.e1–9.

[27] Quintero RA, Chmait RH, Murakoshi T, et al. Surgical management of twin reversed arterial perfusion sequence. Am J Obstet Gynecol 2006;194(4):982–91.

[28] Tan TY, Sepulveda W. Acardiac twin: a systematic review of minimally invasive treatment modalities. Ultrasound Obstet Gynecol 2003;22(4):409–19.

[29] Klaritsch P, Albert K, Van Mieghem T, et al. Instrumental requirements for minimal invasive fetal surgery. BJOG 2008;116(2):188–97.

[30] Lim F, Crombleholme TM, Hedrick HL, et al. Congenital high airway obstruction syndrome: natural history and management. J Pediatr Surg 2003;38(6):940–5.

[31] Liechty KW, Crombleholme TM, Flake AW, et al. Intrapartum airway management for giant fetal neck masses: the EXIT (ex utero intrapartum treatment) procedure. Am J Obstet Gynecol 1997;177(4):870–4.

[32] Mong A, Johnson AM, Kramer SS, et al. Congenital high airway obstruction syndrome: MR/US findings, effect on management, and outcome. Pediatr Radiol 2008;38(11): 1171–9.

[33] Kohl T, Van de Vondel P, Stressig R, et al. Percutaneous fetoscopic laser decompression of congenital high airway obstruction syndrome (CHAOS) from laryngeal atresia via a single trocar–current technical constraints and potential solutions for future interventions. Fetal Diagn Ther 2009;25(1):67–71.

[34] Tran KM, Johnson MP, Almeida-Chen GM, et al. The fetus as patient. Anesthesiology 2010;113(2):462.

[35] Harrison MR, Keller RL, Hawgood SB, et al. A randomized trial of fetal endoscopic tracheal occlusion for severe fetal congenital diaphragmatic hernia. N Engl J Med 2003;349(20): 1916–24.

[36] Deprest JA, Flemmer AW, Gratacos E, et al. Antenatal prediction of lung volume and in-utero treatment by fetal endoscopic tracheal occlusion in severe isolated congenital diaphragmatic hernia. Semin Fetal Neonatal Med 2009;14(1):8–13.

[37] Tworetzky W. Balloon dilation of severe aortic stenosis in the fetus: potential for prevention of hypoplastic left heart syndrome: candidate selection, technique, and results of successful intervention. Circulation 2004;110(15):2125–31.

[38] Makikallio K. Fetal aortic valve stenosis and the evolution of hypoplastic left heart syndrome: patient selection for fetal intervention. Circulation 2006;113(11):1401–5.

[39] Marshall AC, Levine J, Morash D, et al. Results of in uteroatrial septoplasty in fetuses with hypoplastic left heart syndrome. Prenat Diagn 2008;28(11):1023–8.

[40] Tworetzky W, Marshall AC. Fetal interventions for cardiac defects. Pediatr Clin North Am 2004;51(6):1503–13, vii.

[41] Bruner JP, Davis G, Tulipan N. Intrauterine shunt for obstructive hydrocephalus—still not ready. Fetal Diagn Ther 2006;21(6):532–9.

[42] Meuli M, Meuli-Simmen C, Yingling CD, et al. Creation of myelomeningocele in utero: a model of functional damage from spinal cord exposure in fetal sheep. J Pediatr Surg 1995;30(7):1028–32 [discussion: 1032–3].

[43] Meuli M, Meuli-Simmen C, Yingling CD, et al. In utero repair of experimental myelomeningocele saves neurologic function at birth. J Pediatr Surg 1996;31(3):397–402.

[44] Meuli M, Meuli-Simmen C, Hutchins GM, et al. The spinal cord lesion in human fetuses with myelomeningocele: implications for fetal surgery. J Pediatr Surg 1997;32(3):448–52.

[45] Cendron M, D'Alton ME, Crombleholme TM. Prenatal diagnosis and management of the fetus with hydronephrosis. Semin Perinatol 1994;18(3):163–81.

[46] Crombleholme TM, Harrison MR, Langer JC, et al. Early experience with open fetal surgery for congenital hydronephrosis. J Pediatr Surg 1988;23(12):1114–21.

[47] Adzick NS, Crombleholme TM, Morgan MA, et al. A rapidly growing fetal teratoma. Lancet 1997;349(9051):538.

[48] Ibrahim D. Newborn with an open posterior hip dislocation and sciatic nerve injury after intrauterine radiofrequency ablation of a sacrococcygeal teratoma. J Pediatr Surg 2003;38(2):248–50.

[49] Hedrick HL, Flake AW, Crombleholme TM, et al. Sacrococcygeal teratoma: prenatal assessment, fetal intervention, and outcome. J Pediatr Surg 2004;39(3):430–8 [discussion: 430–8].

[50] Tran KM, Flake AW, Kalawadia NV, et al. Emergent excision of a prenatally diagnosed sacrococcygeal teratoma. Paediatr Anaesth 2008;18(5):431–4.

[51] Gin T, Chan MT. Decreased minimum alveolar concentration of isoflurane in pregnant humans. Anesthesiology 1994;81(4):829–32.

[52] Myers LB, Cohen D, Galinkin J, et al. Anaesthesia for fetal surgery. Paediatr Anaesth 2002;12(7):569–78.

[53] Tran KM. Anesthesia for fetal surgery. Semin Fetal Neonatal Med 2010;15(1):40–5.

[54] Myers LB, Bulich LA, Hess P, et al. Fetal endoscopic surgery: indications and anaesthetic management. Best Pract Res Clin Anaesthesiol 2004;18(2):231–58.

[55] Ulmsten U, Sundström G. Esophageal manometry in pregnant and nonpregnant women. Am J Obstet Gynecol 1978;132(3):260–4.

[56] Cormack RS, Lehane J. Difficult tracheal intubation in obstetrics. Anaesthesia 1984;39(11):1105–11.

[57] Samsoon GL, Young JR. Difficult tracheal intubation: a retrospective study. Anaesthesia 1987;42(5):487–90.

[58] Pilkington S, Carli F, Dakin MJ, et al. Increase in Mallampati score during pregnancy. Br J Anaesth 1995;74(6):638–42.

[59] Alaily AB, Carrol KB. Pulmonary ventilation in pregnancy. Br J Obstet Gynaecol 1978;85(7):518–24.

[60] Laird-Meeter K, van de Ley G, Bom TH, et al. Cardiocirculatory adjustments during pregnancy—an echocardiographic study. Clin Cardiol 1979;2(5):328–32.

[61] Motoyama EK, Rivard G, Acheson F, et al. Adverse effect of maternal hyperventilation on the foetus. Lancet 1966;1(7432):286–8.

[62] Motoyama EK, Rivard G, Acheson F, et al. The effect of changes in maternal pH and P-CO$_2$ on the P-O$_2$ of fetal lambs. Anesthesiology 1967;28(5):891–903.

[63] Peng AT, Blancato LS, Motoyama EK. Effect of maternal hypocapnia v. eucapnia on the foetus during Caesarean section. Br J Anaesth 1972;44(11):1173–8.

[64] Palahniuk RJ, Shnider SM. Maternal and fetal cardiovascular and acid-base changes during halothane and isoflurane anesthesia in the pregnant ewe. Anesthesiology 1974;41(5):462–72.

[65] Alahuhta S, Räsänen J, Jouppila R, et al. Effects of extradural bupivacaine with adrenaline for caesarean section on uteroplacental and fetal circulation. Br J Anaesth 1991;67(6):678–82.

[66] Koren G, Pastuszak A, Ito S. Drugs in pregnancy. N Engl J Med 1998;338(16):1128–37.

[67] Sanders RD, Davidson A. Anesthetic-induced neurotoxicity of the neonate: time for clinical guidelines? Paediatr Anaesth 2009;19:1141–6.

[68] Lee SJ, Ralston HJ, Drey EA, et al. Fetal pain: a systematic multidisciplinary review of the evidence. JAMA 2005;294(8):947–54.

[69] Bartocci M, Bergqvist LL, Lagercrantz H, et al. Pain activates cortical areas in the preterm newborn brain. Pain 2006;122(1–2):109–17.

[70] Jevtovic-Todorovic V, Hartman RE, Izumi Y, et al. Early exposure to common anesthetic agents causes widespread neurodegeneration in the developing rat brain and persistent learning deficits. J Neurosci 2003;23(3):876–82.

[71] Istaphanous GK, Loepke AW. General anesthetics and the developing brain. Curr Opin Anaesthesiol 2009;22(3):368–73.

[72] Anand KJ, Aranda JV, Berde CB, et al. Summary proceedings from the neonatal pain-control group. Pediatrics 2006;117:S9–22.

[73] Derbyshire SW. Can fetuses feel pain? BMJ 2006;332(7546):909–12.

[74] Fisk NM, Gitau R, Teixeira JM, et al. Effect of direct fetal opioid analgesia on fetal hormonal and hemodynamic stress response to intrauterine needling. Anesthesiology 2001;95(4): 828–35.

[75] Szwast A, Rychik J. Current concepts in fetal cardiovascular disease. Clin Perinatol 2005;32(4):857–75, viii.

[76] Rychik J. Fetal cardiovascular physiology. Pediatr Cardiol 2004;25(3):1–9.

[77] Morris JA, Hustead RF, Robinson RG, et al. Measurement of fetoplacental blood volume in the human previable fetus. Am J Obstet Gynecol 1974;118(7):927–34.

[78] Nicolaides KH, Clewell WH, Rodeck CH. Measurement of human fetoplacental blood volume in erythroblastosis fetalis. Am J Obstet Gynecol 1987;157(1):50–3.

[79] Reverdiau-Moalic P, Delahousse B, Body G, et al. Evolution of blood coagulation activators and inhibitors in the healthy human fetus. Blood 1996;88(3):900–6.

[80] Gunn TR, Ball KT, Gluckman PD. Reversible umbilical cord occlusion: effects on thermogenesis in utero. Pediatr Res 1991;30(6):513–7.

[81] Marshall AC, Tworetzky W, Bergersen L, et al. Aortic valvuloplasty in the fetus: technical characteristics of successful balloon dilation. J Pediatr 2005;147(4):535–9.

[82] Thaler I, Manor D, Itskovitz J, et al. Changes in uterine blood flow during human pregnancy. Am J Obstet Gynecol 1990;162(1):121–5.

[83] Cullen BF, Margolis AJ, Eger EI. The effects of anesthesia and pulmonary ventilation on blood loss during elective therapeutic abortion. Anesthesiology 1970;32(2):108–13.

[84] Clark KD, Viscomi CM, Lowell J, et al. Nitroglycerin for relaxation to establish a fetal airway (EXIT procedure). Obstet Gynecol 2004;103(5 Pt 2):1113–5.

[85] DiFederico EM, Burlingame JM, Kilpatrick SJ, et al. Pulmonary edema in obstetric patients is rapidly resolved except in the presence of infection or of nitroglycerin tocolysis after open fetal surgery. Am J Obstet Gynecol 1998;179(4):925–33.

[86] Rahbar R, Vogel A, Myers LB, et al. Fetal surgery in otolaryngology: a new era in the diagnosis and management of fetal airway obstruction because of advances in prenatal imaging. Arch Otolaryngol Head Neck Surg 2005;131(5):393–8.

[87] Kunisaki SM, Fauza DO, Barnewolt CE, et al. Ex utero intrapartum treatment with placement on extracorporeal membrane oxygenation for fetal thoracic masses. J Pediatr Surg 2007;42(2):420–5.

[88] Helwig JT, Parer JT, Kilpatrick SJ, et al. Umbilical cord blood acid-base state: what is normal? Am J Obstet Gynecol 1996;174(6):1807–12 [discussion: 1812–4].

Advances in Anesthesia 29 (2011) 149–171

ADVANCES IN ANESTHESIA

ELSEVIER
MOSBY

Clinical Pathways for Total Joint Arthroplasty: Essential Components for Success

Rebecca L. Johnson, MD, Christopher M. Duncan, MD, James R. Hebl, MD*

Department of Anesthesiology, Mayo Clinic College of Medicine, 200 First Street Southwest, Rochester, MN 55905, USA

CLINICAL PATHWAYS: AN OVERVIEW

The term, *clinical pathway*, refers to a multidisciplinary process of mutual decision making that results in the organized care of a well-defined group of patients during a well-defined period of time [1,2]. Clinical pathways were first introduced in the 1980s when escalating medical costs pressured physicians to decrease resource use without jeopardizing patient safety or clinical outcomes. At that time, pathways were typically procedure specific (eg, coronary artery bypass grafting, total knee arthroplasty) and tailored to a specific institution [3,4]. As a result, tremendous variability often existed from one institutional clinical pathway to another, making clinical comparisons between pathways and formal scientific study difficult.

Despite this variability, it is generally agreed that clinical pathways provide several distinct advantages. These include the ability to (1) provide coordinated care between departments and across patient care units, (2) standardize patient care and reduce hospital length-of-stay, (3) convert typical inpatient (ie, same-day admission) procedures to outpatient (ie, same-day discharge) procedures, (4) prompt change in the care process to better emphasize patient outcomes and cost containment, (5) control hospital costs, and (6) serve as a marketing tool with the public or with third-party payers [5].

In contrast, major limitations of clinical pathways include the inability to share and compare clinical advances that are often generated from newly implemented pathways. Sharing information is difficult because of the lack of scientific rigor (ie, clinical outcomes are often analyzed retrospectively and compared with historical controls) and the absence of guidelines or recommendations on how

Financial support: Mayo Clinic Department of Anesthesiology.
Financial disclosure: The authors have nothing to disclose.

*Corresponding author. E-mail address: hebl.james@mayo.edu

0737-6146/11/$ – see front matter
doi:10.1016/j.aan.2011.08.001

best to describe clinical pathway processes and associated outcome data within scientific journals [5]. Comparison of information is difficult because of the precise nature in which clinical pathways are developed. Most clinical pathways are large multidisciplinary projects from high-volume institutions that attempt to standardize health care processes for a predefined patient population within a single hospital or clinic based on current processes, clinical outcomes, and the unique preferences of participating health care professionals. This process of development (which is a benefit for the participating institution) makes widespread application to other institutions (with their own unique processes, outcomes, and preferences) difficult [5]. Variables that often differ from one published clinical pathway to another—and thus make clinical comparisons difficult— are listed in Box 1.

Despite these challenges, this review summarizes the important components of a successful clinical pathway and attempts to evaluate the impact of differing clinical pathways on major perioperative outcomes after total joint arthroplasty. Perioperative outcomes evaluated include postoperative complications, hospital length-of-stay, clinical outcomes, and medical costs.

CLINICAL PATHWAY COMPONENTS

Effective clinical pathways for major orthopedic surgery include the coordination and standardization of several patient care activities during the preoperative, intraoperative, and postoperative period. Essential components of some of the most effective orthopedic clinical pathways are listed in Box 2.

Preoperative patient education

Major orthopedic surgery can be a stressful and anxiety-provoking experience for most patients. Bondy and colleagues [6] examined the effect of anesthesia patient education on preoperative anxiety and found that a detailed patient education program may have several beneficial effects. Preoperative patient education may significantly relieve patient anxiety and emotional stress by providing a better understanding of the perioperative process (eg, preoperative evaluation, hospital admission process, anesthetic options, and expected clinical course) and establishing clear expectations with regard to hospital length-of-stay and the discharge process (eg, dismissal to home vs rehabilitation swing-bed vs nursing home). Because patients have a better understanding of the perioperative process, they often present for surgery with increased confidence in the therapeutic plan and a willingness to more actively participate in their care. Increased participation often results in greater patient satisfaction and potentially improved perioperative outcomes. The extent to which patient education influences postoperative outcomes, however, is somewhat unclear [7–9]. McDonald and colleagues [8] demonstrated that preoperative patient education may result in a modest benefit in preoperative anxiety. This benefit failed to persist, however, on postoperative day (POD) 2 or at the time of hospital discharge. A review of the Cochrane Database on this topic fails to demonstrate that preoperative patient education has a significant impact on postoperative

Box 1: Clinical pathway variables

Patient population
- Age restrictions
- Gender
- Body mass index limitations
- Comorbid patient conditions

Surgical variables
- Minimally invasive versus traditional surgical approaches
- Mini-incision versus standard incision
- Surgical approach (anterior vs posterior)

Clinical pathway interventions
- Preoperative
  - Patient education classes
  - Preoperative medical evaluations
  - Preoperative medical management of psychiatric conditions (eg, anxiety, depression, and pain)
  - Preoperative oral multimodal analgesic regimen
- Intraoperative
  - General anesthesia
  - Neuraxial anesthesia (spinal vs epidural anesthesia)
  - Peripheral nerve blockade only
- Postoperative
  - Oral versus intravenous opioids
  - Use of nonopioid adjuvant therapy (multimodal regimen)
  - Continuous neuraxial catheters
  - Continuous peripheral nerve catheters
  - Physical therapy regimen

Study definitions and outcome assessments
- Pain scores (pain assessments at rest vs with activity vs both)
- Opioid requirements
- Opioid-related side effects (variable definitions)
- Rehabilitation outcomes (variable definitions of rehabilitation milestones)
- Postoperative complications (variable definitions)
- Discharge eligibility (variable definitions)
- Hospital length-of-stay
- Costs (total costs vs direct costs)

Box 2: Essential clinical pathway components

Preoperative
- Preoperative patient education program
- Appropriate management of preoperative pain and psychological symptoms (fear, anxiety, and depression)

Intraoperative
- Development of a comprehensive multimodal analgesic regimen
- The use of peripheral nerve blockade and continuous perineural catheters
- Postanesthesia care unit (PACU) algorithms for the management of acute postoperative pain

Postoperative
- Standardized method of pain assessment on the nursing floors and pain score documentation within the medical record
- Early and accelerated rehabilitation regimen
- Development of an integrated and multidisciplinary acute pain service
- Staff education regarding the importance of pain management
- Written protocols for acute postoperative pain management

---

clinical outcomes (eg, postoperative pain, functional outcomes, hospital length-of-stay) in patients undergoing total hip or total knee arthroplasty.

Multimodal analgesia

Patients undergoing total knee and total hip arthroplasty experience significant postoperative pain [10]. Severe pain occurs in 60% of patients and moderate pain in up to 30% of patients undergoing total knee arthroplasty. Failure to provide adequate analgesia may impede early physical therapy and rapid rehabilitation [11], which are both important factors for maintaining joint range of motion and facilitating hospital discharge [12]. In an effort to avoid many of the side effects commonly associated with opioid-induced analgesia, clinicians have begun adopting multimodal therapeutic regimens. Multimodal analgesia has become an important concept in the field of modern pain management [12–17]. The concept is designed to combat pain perception along several pathways of signal transmission, including the surgical site and surrounding tissues, local sensory nerves, and central nervous system. Advantages include superior analgesia secondary to the synergistic effects of multiple agents acting via different pathways, the ability to limit parenteral opioid administration, and minimizing opioid-related side effects. Several investigations have demonstrated the beneficial effects of multimodal analgesia [14–16], including its value in patients undergoing major orthopedic joint replacement surgery [17–24].

Several medications may be used as part of a multimodal analgesic pathway. Specifically, the use of acetaminophen [25], nonsteroidal anti-inflammatory agents [26], selective cyclooxygenase (COX)-2 inhibitors inhibitors [18], prega-balin [21], and ketamine [22] has been shown to have analgesic benefits in patients undergoing joint replacement surgery. Most experts recommend using multiple agents during the preoperative and postoperative period in small quantitative doses to maximize the analgesic effect while minimizing associated side effects. Documented benefits include superior postoperative analgesia [18,22,25,26], reduced supplemental opioid requirements [18,21,22,25,26], fewer opioid-related side effects [13,18], improved joint range of motion [18,21], fewer postoperative sleep disturbances [18], shorter time to achieve hospital discharge criteria [21], improved functional mobility [22], and a lower incidence of chronic neuropathic pain [21].

Finally, poorly controlled acute postoperative (ie, nociceptive) pain may contribute to the development of chronic neuropathic pain or complex regional pain syndrome after total joint arthroplasty [27]. Nikolajsen and colleagues [28] examined the Danish Hip Arthroplasty Registry and found that 12% of patients continue to experience moderate-to-severe pain 12 to 18 months after surgery. Similarly, up to 13% of total knee arthroplasty patients may experience moderate-to-severe pain 12-months after surgery [29]. Additional risk factors for the development of chronic postoperative pain include preoperative pain for greater than 1 month, an increased intensity of preoperative pain, and a patient history of preoperative fear, anxiety, or depression [29,30]. Poorly controlled postoperative pain has also been shown to impede global recovery and lower the reported quality of life 6 months after surgery [31]. Therefore, clinical pathways that integrate (1) a comprehensive multimodal analgesic regimen to adequately manage preoperative and postoperative pain and (2) a comprehensive psychiatric program to manage preoperative psychological symptoms may have a significant benefit in improving long-term clinical and psychiatric outcomes.

Peripheral nerve blockade and continuous perineural catheters

Many treatment regimens for managing severe postoperative orthopedic pain include significant doses of parenteral opioids. These treatment regimens are commonly associated with significant opioid-related side effects, such as seda-tion, nausea, vomiting, ileus, and urinary retention, that can adversely effect patient outcomes and prolong hospital length-of-stay [19]. Therefore, clinical pathways that minimize (or eliminate) opioid administration may significantly reduce opioid-related side effects and improve postoperative patient outcomes.

The integration of regional anesthesia and peripheral nerve blockade into clinical pathways for orthopedic surgery is an essential step to minimize opioid use and improve perioperative outcomes. Both single-injection [32–35] and continuous [36–40] peripheral nerve block techniques have been shown to provide superior analgesia, reduce supplemental opioid requirements, decrease opioid-related side effects, and improve functional outcomes after total joint ar-throplasty. In a recent meta-analysis of 19 articles and 603 patients, Richman and colleagues [41] demonstrated that patients receiving continuous peripheral nerve blockade have superior analgesia, fewer opioid-related side effects (nausea, vomiting, pruritus, and sedation), and improved patient satisfaction compared with traditional intravenous opioids alone. Although single-injection techniques have been shown to be superior to placebo or systemic analgesia [32–35], comparison studies have shown that single-injection blocks fail to provide the extended benefits of continuous perineural catheters [37,42,43]. Continuous peripheral nerve block techniques have also been shown to have similar analgesia—but a more desirable side effect profile—compared with epidural analgesia [44]. A recent review by Fowler and colleagues [44] demonstrated that patients receiving peripheral nerve blocks had less urinary retention and fewer episodes of postoperative hypotension compared with patients receiving neuraxial techniques.

A primary concern regarding the use of peripheral nerve blockade is the risk of neurologic complications. Barrington and colleagues [45] recently performed a prospective audit of more than 7000 peripheral nerve blocks performed at 9 Australian hospitals. Overall, they identified a neurologic injury rate of 0.5%. Only 10% of these injuries were attributed to peripheral nerve blockade, however, suggesting that the majority of perioperative nerve injuries have a nonanesthesia-related cause. The nerve injury rate attributed to peripheral nerve blockade was 0.04%—a rate similar to that in other large-scale investigations [46,47]. Jacob and colleagues [48] also demonstrated that neither the type of intraoperative anesthesia (general vs neuraxial) nor the use of peripheral nerve blockade was associated with an increased risk of perioperative nerve injury in 12,329 patients undergoing total knee arthroplasty. Rather, bilateral surgical procedures and total tourniquet time were found associated with an increased risk of nerve injury [48].

Standardized pain assessment and documentation, pain management protocols and staff education

In 2001, the Joint Commission declared pain the fifth vital sign and instituted pain management standards for accredited ambulatory care facilities, behavioral health care organizations, critical access hospitals, home care providers, hospitals, office-based surgery practices, and long-term care providers [49]. The standard requires health care providers to (1) appropriately assess and manage pain, (2) document pain management interventions and subsequent reassessments, (3) perform pain screenings during initial patient assessments, and (4) educate patients and their families about pain management. Benhamou and colleagues [50] and Fletcher and colleagues [51] report that similar guidelines and recommendations have been put forward by the Royal College of Surgeons, the French Ministry of Health, the French Society of Anesthesia and Intensive Care, the European Task Force on Pain Management, and the International Association for the Study of Pain. The overwhelming consensus is that each of these interventions should be considered essential components to any clinical pathway designed to optimize pain management and patient care.

Despite these recommendations, the literature suggests that pain remains undertreated in both US [52] and European [53] health care facilities—in part because of a lack of adherence to previously published standards and guidelines. Benhamou and colleagues [50] recently surveyed 746 hospitals in 7 European countries and identified major deficiencies in postoperative pain management. Specifically,

- 34% of respondents stated that pain is not routinely assessed.
- 56% of respondents stated that pain scores are not documented in the patient's medical record.
- 75% of respondents stated that they do not have written postoperative pain management protocols.
- 52% of respondents stated that they do not routinely provide patients with information on postoperative pain management.
- 34% of respondents do not have regular on-site staff training programs on postoperative pain management.

Recent efforts by the French Ministry of Health, professional nursing organizations, and local hospitals to improve pain management in France have resulted in significant progress in many health care facilities. In a survey of 76 French surgical centers, 94% of respondents stated that pain is routinely assessed and documented within the medical record (every 4 hours) and that 74% of centers have standardized postoperative pain protocols [51]. These and other improvements are only possible when pain is routinely assessed and documented within the medical record. Many hospitals are performing local audits to ensure compliance with institutional standards while educating health care staff on the importance of pain management strategies [54].

Early and accelerated rehabilitation

An early and accelerated rehabilitation program should also be integrated into clinical pathways designed for total hip and total knee arthroplasty patients. A review of the literature suggests that early and accelerated rehabilitation may have a major impact on improved perioperative outcomes in orthopedic patients [9,55]. Munin and colleagues [55] demonstrated that early inpatient rehabilitation resulted in a shorter hospital length-of-stay and a more rapid attainment of short-term functional outcomes after joint replacement surgery compared with a delayed rehabilitation program. Pour and colleagues [9] also examined the impact of an accelerated preoperative and postoperative rehabilitation program versus a standard regimen on functional outcomes after total hip arthroplasty. Patients randomized to the accelerated pathway were seen earlier on the day of surgery and more frequently on subsequent PODs (twice daily vs once daily). There was also a greater emphasis on oral analgesics (vs intravenous patient-controlled analgesia) in patients receiving accelerated rehabilitation. In addition to a shorter hospital length-of-stay, accelerated pathway patients were able to walk for longer distances, had improved pain control, and reported higher patient satisfaction at the time of hospital discharge [9].

Finally, Mahomed and colleagues [56] have demonstrated that rehabilitation after total hip or total knee arthroplasty does not need to be restricted to the inpatient setting. Home-based rehabilitation programs may provide similar degrees of postoperative analgesia, functional outcomes, and patient satisfaction at a significantly lower cost compared with hospital-based regimens [56].

CLINICAL PATHWAYS AND PERIOPERATIVE OUTCOMES

The goal of most clinical pathways is to provide standardized, evidence-based care to patients in such a way as to minimize the variability of care provided by individual providers. This process has the potential to significantly enhance the quality, improve the safety, and reduce the cost associated with surgical procedures. Several clinical pathways have been reported in the literature for patients undergoing total joint arthroplasty [1,4,19,20,57–59], with no two pathways identical. As a result, comparison of clinical pathways is difficult—forcing systematic reviews or meta-analyses that examine the topic to comment on the concept of clinical pathways versus their individual component parts. Barbieri and colleagues [1] recently performed a systematic review of clinical pathways used for joint replacement surgery. The review examined 22 studies and included 6316 patients. The aggregate results demonstrated a significant reduction in postoperative complications (deep venous thrombosis, pulmonary embolism, manipulation, superficial infection, deep infection, and heel decubitus ulcers), a shorter hospital length-of-stay, and lower hospital costs in patients undergoing clinical pathways versus standard care [1]. Publications from the University of California, Irvine; the University of Utah; and the Mayo Clinic are discussed below and represent typical examples of clinical pathways developed for orthopedic surgical patients.

Skinner and Shintani [57] performed a retrospective, case-controlled investigation of 102 patients undergoing total hip or total knee arthroplasty at the University of California, Irvine. They compared a multimodal clinical pathway that incorporated COX-2 inhibitors, tramadol, dexamethasone, acetaminophen, and intra-articular bupivacaine with standard management of patient-controlled analgesia and intravenous opioids. The investigators did not incorporate regional anesthesia or peripheral nerve blockade as a component of the clinical pathway. Clinical endpoints were evaluated during PODs 1 through 4. For patients receiving the clinical pathway, opioid requirements were reduced 66% for total hip arthroplasty (POD 2 only) and 68% for total knee arthroplasty (POD 3 only). Although verbal analog scale (VAS) pain scores were no different among total hip arthroplasty patients, patients undergoing total knee arthroplasty reported lower VAS pain scores on POD 2 and at the time of hospital discharge. Implementation of the clinical pathway resulted in no differences in perioperative complications. Hospital length-of-stay was reduced in only total knee arthroplasty patients undergoing the clinical pathway (4.0 vs 4.9 days; $P<.02$) [57].

In contrast to clinical pathways not incorporating regional anesthesia [57], multimodal regimens using peripheral nerve blockade have been shown to consistently reduce hospital length-of-stay, improve perioperative analgesia with fewer opioid medications, facilitate postoperative rehabilitation, and reduce opioid-related side effects [19,20,58]. Peters and colleagues [58] performed a retrospective analysis of 100 patients undergoing total hip and total knee arthroplasty at the University of Utah. The clinical pathway included a multimodal analgesic regimen (sustained-release oxycodone, COX-2 inhibitors, and acetaminophen), intraoperative regional anesthesia with intrathecal opioids, and an ultrasound-guided femoral nerve catheter (total knee arthroplasty patients only) for extended postoperative analgesia. Before wound closure, patients undergoing both total hip and total knee arthroplasty received less than 1 mg/kg of 0.25% bupivacaine injected into the deep and subcutaneous tissues by the orthopedic surgeon. A multimodal oral analgesic regimen was then continued into the postoperative period. Control patients were managed with intraoperative general or spinal anesthesia (with intrathecal morphine), continuous femoral nerve blockade (total knee arthroplasty patients only), and postoperative patient-controlled analgesia with intravenous opioids. Patients receiving the clinical pathway had significantly lower pain scores at rest on PODs 1 and 2, lower opioid requirements, improved ambulation during rehabilitation sessions, and reduced hospital length-of-stay. There were no differences in perioperative complications when comparing clinical pathway with control patients. Overall, the investigators concluded that development and implementation of a comprehensive clinical pathway combined with early and aggressive physical therapy improve perioperative outcomes, shorten hospital length-of-stay, and allow patients to achieved physical therapy goals earlier compared with nonclinical pathway patients [58].

Finally, Hebl and colleagues have described the development and implementation of the Mayo Clinic Total Joint Regional Anesthesia (TJRA) Clinical Pathway in patients undergoing both minimally invasive [19] and traditional [20] total hip and total knee arthroplasty. The TJRA Clinical Pathway incorporates preoperative patient education, a multimodal analgesic regimen emphasizing peripheral nerve blockade, standardized PACU algorithms, pain assessments and medical record documentation, pain management protocols, and a standardized postoperative physical therapy regimen for patients undergoing total joint arthroplasty. Similar to most clinical pathways, the TJRA Clinical Pathway was developed by a multidisciplinary group of Mayo Clinic surgeons, anesthesiologists, pharmacists, nurses, and physical therapy staff based on their collective experience and exposure to physicians and practice models outside the institution. Although the basic principles of the pathway have remained unchanged (eg, preoperative patient education, multimodal analgesia, peripheral nerve blockade, pain management protocols), its individual components are continually being evaluated and modified as necessary based on changes in clinical practice. The current multimodal analgesic and regional anesthesia components of the TJRA Clinical Pathway are listed in Box 3.

The Mayo Clinic TJRA Clinical Pathway was first used in patients undergoing minimally invasive total hip (n = 20) and total knee (n = 20) arthroplasty [19]. Study patients were prospectively enrolled and compared with matched historical controls undergoing traditional surgical and anesthetic techniques. Matching

Box 3: Mayo Clinic Total Joint Regional Anesthesia Clinical Pathway[a]

Patient waiting area (preoperative)

- Oxycodone controlled release (OxyContin), 20 mg po, once on arrival to patient waiting area if patient 18 to 59 years old, or 10 mg po, if patient 60 to 74 years old
- Acetaminophen (Tylenol), 1000 mg po, once on arrival to patient waiting area
- Celecoxib (Celebrex), 400 mg po, once on arrival to patient waiting area
- Gabapentin (Neurontin), 600 mg po, once on arrival to patient waiting area if patient is 18 to 59 years old, or 300 mg po, if patient 60 to 69 years old

Peripheral nerve catheter infusions

- Femoral catheters (total knee arthroplasty)
  - Bupivacaine, 0.2% 10 mL bolus, on arrival in PACU, then initiate continuous infusion bupivacaine, 0.2% at 10 mL/h
  - Continue bupivacaine, 0.2% continuous infusion at 10 mL/h, until 0600 the day after surgery. At 0600 the day after surgery, change to bupivacaine, 0.1% continuous infusion at 10 mL/h. On the second day after surgery, stop infusion and discontinue femoral nerve catheter infusion before 0800.
- Posterior lumbar plexus catheters (total hip arthroplasty)
  - Bupivacaine, 0.2% 10 mL bolus, on arrival in PACU, then initiate continuous infusion bupivacaine, 0.2% at 10 mL/h
  - Continue bupivacaine, 0.2% continuous infusion at 10 mL/h, until 0600 the day after surgery. At 0600 the day after surgery, change to bupivacaine, 0.1% continuous infusion at 10 mL/h. On the second day after surgery, stop infusion and discontinue psoas nerve catheter infusion before 0800.

PACU

- Oxycodone, 5 mg to 10 mg po prn, once for pain rated 4 or greater. Give 5 mg if patient 70 years old or older; give 10 mg if patient 18 to 69 years old.
- Fentanyl, 25 µg intravenous prn, for pain rated 7 or greater; may repeat every 5 minutes (maximum 100 µg)
- Ketorolac (Toradol), 15 mg intravenous prn, once for pain rated 4 or greater

Postoperative nursing floor[b]

- Acetaminophen (Tylenol), 1000 mg po 3 times daily at 0800, 1200, and 1600 hours.
- Tramadol (Ultram), 50 mg to 100 mg po every 6 hours
- Celecoxib (Celebrex), 200 mg po bid
- Ketorolac (Toradol), 15 mg intravenous every 6 hours prn, for pain rated more than 4 (maximum of 4 doses)
- Oxycodone, 5 mg to 10 mg po every 4 hours prn. Give 5 mg if patient reports pain and rates pain score less than 4; give 10 mg if patient complains of pain rated 4 or greater.

Monitoring

- Continuous pulse oximetry for 48 hours postoperatively

[a]Perioperative analgesic options are selected based on each patient's associated comorbidities.
[b]Selection of postoperative medications at surgeon's discretion.

criteria included the type of surgical procedure, age, gender, and American Society of Anesthesiologists physical status (ASA-PS) classification. Patients undergoing minimally invasive surgery in combination with the TJRA Clinical Pathway had significantly lower pain scores both at rest and with physical therapy, required fewer opioid medications, were able to ambulate significantly sooner, and experienced less urinary retention and postoperative cognitive dysfunction compared with matched controls. Cognitive dysfunction was defined as disorientation to person, place, or time, hallucinations, or any other cognitive condition requiring further assessment by a physician. Based on these criteria, approximately 15% of control patients and 1% of TJRA patients experience postoperative cognitive dysfunction during their hospitalization. Hospital length-of-stay was also significantly shorter among TJRA patients (2.8 days vs 5.0 days; $P<.01$) [19].

The Mayo Clinic TJRA Clinical Pathways has also been used in patients undergoing traditional (ie, nonminimally invasive) total hip and total knee arthroplasty [20]. Patients undergoing joint replacement surgery with the TJRA Clinical Pathway experience superior analgesia with fewer opioid-related side effects compared with control patients. VAS pain scores were significantly lower among TJRA patients both at rest ($P<.001$) and with activity ($P<.001$) during their entire hospital stay. Opioid requirements were significantly less among TJRA patients from the preoperative/intraoperative period until the beginning of POD 2 ($P=.04$). Opioid-related side effects, such as nausea ($P<.001$), vomiting ($P=.01$), and urinary retention ($P<.001$), were also significantly reduced for TJRA patients throughout most of the perioperative period. There was no significant difference in the frequency of pruritus between groups [20].

Postoperative milestones (bed-to-chair transfer, discharge eligibility, and hospital dismissal) were achieved significantly sooner in patients receiving the multimodal TJRA protocol. The ability to transfer from bed to chair occurs a mean of 0.2 ± 0.6 days sooner among TJRA patients compared with matched controls ($P=.001$). Nearly all patients, however, were able to accomplish this milestone by the end of POD 1. Discharge eligibility was also achieved a mean of 1.7 ± 1.9 days sooner among TJRA patients compared with matched controls ($P<.0001$). Hospital length-of-stay was 3.8 days for TJRA patients and 5.0 days for controls ($P<.001$). At the time of hospital dismissal, joint range of motion was significantly better among TJRA patients ($90°$ vs $85°$; $P=.008$). The small gains in range of motion observed at hospital dismissal persisted at 6 to 8 weeks postoperatively ($106°$ vs $99°$; $P=.03$) [20].

Severe postoperative complications (neurologic injury, myocardial infarction, renal dysfunction, localized bleeding, deep venous thrombosis/pulmonary embolism, joint dislocation, and wound infection) were similar among TJRA patients and patients receiving patient-controlled analgesia. Urinary retention ($P<.001$) and postoperative ileus occurred significantly more often among control patients (7% vs 1%; $P=.01$) resulting in delayed postoperative feedings [20].

CLINICAL PATHWAYS AND ECONOMIC OUTCOMES

Total hip and total knee arthroplasty are two of the most commonly performed surgical procedures in the United States and represent the single greatest Medicare procedural expenditure [60,61]. Recent data from the United States Healthcare Cost and Utilization Project report that both the number and cost of total knee and total hip replacement surgeries have increased more than 300% during the past decade [62,63]. Furthermore, the American Academy of Orthopaedic Surgeons and other independent population-based studies estimate that the number of total joint replacement surgeries will continue to grow [64,65]. The number of total hip arthroplasties is expected to increase by as much as 50% per year and the number of total knee arthroplasties by 300% per year through the year 2030 [64]. Given this trend and the fact that Medicare reimbursement continues to decline, orthopedic patients may have a major economic impact on hospitals and other health care facilities during the next 20 years [66]. Therefore, any changes in surgical or anesthetic practice that can reduce the cost associated with these procedures—while maintaining the same degree of high-quality and efficient patient care—may have a significant impact on overall United States health care expenditures.

Medical costs associated with an episode of care can be classified into 3 major categories: (1) indirect costs, (2) intangible costs, and (3) direct costs [67]. Indirect costs include the cost of lost productivity related to the morbidity and mortality of the disease state. Intangible costs include the cost associated with pain and suffering from the disease state. Direct costs include medical supplies, labor, and time—and can be further divided into Medicare Part A costs and Medicare Part B costs (Fig. 1). Several cohort studies have linked the use of clinical pathways with lower variable costs [7,68–74]. Other studies have demonstrated that the development and implementation of a clinical pathway for patients undergoing total hip or total knee arthroplasty may significantly reduce both total hospital [4] and direct medical costs [62] while maintaining or improving perioperative outcomes.

Macario and colleagues [4] examined the impact of implementing a comprehensive clinical pathway on total hospital costs for patients undergoing total knee arthroplasty. The clinical pathway was developed by a multidisciplinary group of providers (orthopedic surgeons, anesthesiologists, nursing, pharmacy, infectious disease and transfusion medicine specialists, and information technology personnel) to standardize the care of patients undergoing elective orthopedic surgery (Box 4). The sum of fixed and variable costs (ie, total hospital costs) were prospectively evaluated from 10 major departments (surgical admissions, operating room, anesthesia, postanesthesia care unit, patient ward, ICU, radiology, pharmacy, laboratory, and blood bank) and compared with historical controls. Overall, the orthopedic clinical pathway reduced hospital costs by 19% ($17,618 vs $21,709). Of the total cost savings, 54% resulted from decreasing operating room costs (decreased operative time and resource use) and 16% resulted from decreasing patient ward costs (decreased hospital length-of-stay). The remaining 30% reduction in costs included decreases in

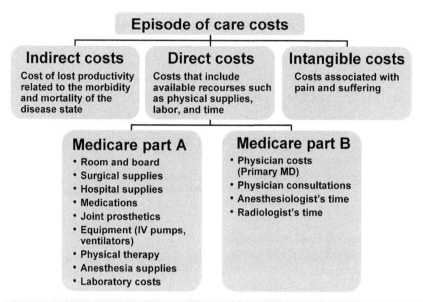

Fig. 1. Classification of episode of care costs.

pharmacy (8%), physical therapy (6%), blood bank (4%), anesthesia (3%), radiology (3%), PACU (2%), and miscellaneous (4%) costs. The investigators speculated that one of the primary advantages of clinical pathways is the ability to reduce the portion of financial risk due to provider variability [4].

Duncan and colleagues [62] have also shown that the implementation of a comprehensive, preemptive multimodal clinical pathway may reduce direct medical costs associated with lower-extremity joint replacement surgery. A detailed economic analysis was performed from the perspective of the health care system. Data from administrative sources were used to evaluate and compare the direct medical costs between the TJRA Clinical Pathway (see Box 3) and control cohorts for each surgical episode of care. Billed charges were grouped into the Medicare Part A and Part B classification system (see Fig. 1). Costs associated with Medicare Part A hospital services were estimated by adjusting billed charges using cost-to-charge ratios at the department level and wage indexes. Costs associated with Medicare Part B physician services were acquired using Medicare reimbursement rates.

The estimated hospital (Medicare Part A), physician (Medicare Part B), and total costs for each cohort are listed in Table 1. Overall, total direct medical costs of hospitalization were $1999 lower for TJRA patients compared with controls ($14,990 vs $16,989; 95% CI, $584–$3231). Component analysis of hospital (Medicare Part A) and physician (Medicare Part B) costs found that hospital-based costs were significantly reduced within the TJRA cohort and accounted for the majority of the total cost savings. The observed difference in hospital costs was attributed primarily to significant reductions in medical

Box 4: Stanford University Medical Center clinical pathway for total knee arthroplasty

Preoperative
- Standardization of preoperative laboratory evaluation
- Standardization of 2 units autologous blood donation

Surgical admission unit
- Intravenous access established by nursing staff
- Epidural catheter insertion by anesthesia staff
- Functioning epidural confirmed before surgical incision
- Standardized antibiotic use and administration

Intraoperative
- Standardized surgical instrumentation
- Standardized total knee arthroplasty surgical supply pack (vs general total joint arthroplasty pack)
- Standardized times established for
  - Room set-up
  - Operating room entry
  - Procedure
  - Turnover
- Autologous blood retrieval system eliminated
- Criteria established for use of reinfusion drains
- Standardization of joint prosthetic implants

PACU
- Standardized order sets
- Standardized times established for length-of-stay
- Standardized discharge criteria established

and surgical supply costs, operating room costs, and anesthesia supply costs. Although room and board and pharmacy costs were also reduced within the TJRA Clinical Pathway cohort, these component costs were not found to be statistically significant. Overall, physician costs (Medicare Part B) were not found to be significantly different between groups.

A subgroup analysis was also performed to evaluate whether or not patient co-morbidities influenced cost savings. The estimated hospital (Medicare Part A), physician (Medicare Part B), and total costs for ASA PS I-II and ASA PS III-IV patients are listed in Table 2. Among ASA I-II patients, the TJRA cohort had significantly lower hospital (Medicare Part A) and overall total costs compared with control patients. Anesthesia physician costs were also significantly lower among TJRA patients. In contrast, ASA III-IV patients within the TJRA cohort

Table 1
Hospital and physician costs of total joint replacement surgery[a]

	TJRA cohort (n = 96)[b]	Control cohort (n = 96)[b]	Cost difference (95% CI$)[c]	P value
Hospital costs (Medicare Part A)	$12,505 ($11,640) ± $4584	$14,415 ($13,126) ± $4532	$1911 ($578–3111)	0.0002
Room and board	$4346 ($3899) ± $1176	$4647 ($4252) ± $1513	$300 (−$84–718)	0.14
Medical and surgical supplies	$2544 ($2036) ± $1572	$3388 ($2784) ± $1733	$844 ($378–1277)	<0.0001
Operating room	$2641 ($2620) ± $389	$3014 ($2969) ± $486	$373 ($246–489)	<0.0001
Pharmacy	$746 ($693) ± $192	$1152 ($786) ± $2161	$406 ($101–876)	0.07
Anesthesia supply	$129 ($177) ± $63	$164 ($212) ± $88	$36 ($14–56)	0.002
Physician costs (Medicare Part B)	$2486 ($2262) ± $683	$2574 ($2526) ± $410	$88 (−$77–239)	0.30
Anesthesia	$368 ($359) ± $61	$444 ($444) ± $78	$76 ($57–95)	<0.0001
Total costs	$14,990 ($14,226) ± $4773	$16,989 ($15,697) ± $4786	$1999 ($584–3231)	0.0004

[a] Estimated costs per patient are reported in 2004 constant dollars.
[b] Values are presented as mean (median) ± SD.
[c] Intrapair differences are calculated as control minus TJRA cohort. Bootstrap 95% CI using the percentile method.

had significantly lower physician costs (Medicare Part B) compared with ASA III-IV controls. Although total costs were also lower among ASA III-IV patients within the TJRA Clinical Pathway, this difference did not reach statistical significance due to greater variability among these patients.

A reduction in hospital length-of-stay is often considered a cost-saving benefit during the perioperative period. Cost savings associated with reductions in hospital length-of-stay, however, are directly related to the total duration of stay and may not necessarily reflect a significant source of cost savings. For example, although hospital room and board costs remain constant throughout a hospitalization, treatment costs associated with a hospitalization are often greatest during the initial 48 to 72 hours of care (reflecting greater care demands during the patient's initial illness), with a subsequent decline in daily direct medical (ie, treatment) costs (Fig. 2) [75]. Therefore, a reduction in hospital length-of-stay from 72 hours to 48 hours results in significantly greater cost savings than a length-of-stay reduction from 7 days to 6 days. As a result, hospital administrators must understand that an isolated reduction in length-of-stay may (or may not) result in a positive financial impact for the hospital or institution.

LIMITATIONS OF CLINICAL PATHWAYS

Effective perioperative pain management is not without potential consequences. In 2001, the Joint Commission on Accreditation of Healthcare Organizations declared pain the fifth vital sign and mandated that pain management become an integral component of all patient care activities as a condition of hospital accreditation. As a result, many institutions implemented aggressive pain management protocols that were guided by patient reports of pain intensity as quantified by a numeric pain scale. Although numeric pains scales may be useful to monitor pain trends within a given patient, these subjective methods of pain assessment are a poor guide for directed analgesic management. Because these subjective and often nonreproducible pain scales do not take into consideration patient co-morbidities or associated medication risks, adverse outcomes such as oversedation and respiratory depression may lead to catastrophic outcomes, including death [70,76,77].

Vila and colleagues [78] demonstrated the potential negative impact of implementing a hospital-wide pain management protocol that treats pain based on patient self-reports. After implementation of a numeric pain treatment algorithm, the number of adverse drug reactions secondary to opioid oversedation more than doubled compared with preimplementation values (24.5 vs 11 adverse events per 100,000 inpatient hospital days; $P<.001$). A decreased level of consciousness preceded 94% of events, emphasizing the importance of careful clinical assessment and ongoing patient monitoring while managing pain [78]. Overmedication in preparation for an imaging study [70], overmedication after discharge from the ICU [70], and the first 24 hours after surgery [77] seem to be the clinical scenarios or time periods in which patients are at greatest risk for respiratory depression and oversedation.

Table 2
Hospital and physician costs of total joint replacement surgery and ASA physical status[a]

ASA I-II patients	TJRA cohort[b] (n = 55)	Control cohort[b] (n = 55)	Cost difference[c] (95% CI$)	P value
Hospital costs (Medicare Part A)	$11,716 ($11,375) ± $2107	$13,454 ($12,536) ± $3583	$1738 ($712–2876)	0.003
Physician costs (Medicare Part B)	$2572 ($2274) ± $809	$2555 ($2526) ± $401	−$16 (−$271–223)	0.89
Anesthesia	$354 ($351) ± $45	$446 ($444) ± $85	$91 ($67–115)	<0.0001
Total costs	$14,288 ($14,083) ± $2395	$16,010 ($15,172) ± $3848	$1722 ($594–2954)	0.006
ASA III-IV patients	**TJRA cohort[b] (n = 38)**	**Control cohort[b] (n = 38)**	**Cost difference[c] (95% CI)**	**P value**
Hospital costs (Medicare Part A)	$13,746 ($12,767) ± $6695	$15,631 ($13,935) ± $5232	$1885 (−$1130–4376)	0.18
Physician costs (Medicare Part B)	$2360 ($2253) ± $419	$2595 ($2566) ± 428	$235 ($47–430)	0.02
Anesthesia	$388 ($361) ± 77	$444 ($446) ± 68	$55 ($22–86)	0.001
Total costs	$16,106 ($14,774) ± $6925	$18,226 ($16,515) ± $5480	$2120 (−$996–4702)	0.14

[a] Estimated costs per patient are reported in 2004 constant dollars.
[b] Values are presented as mean (median) ± SD.
[c] Intrapair differences are calculated as control minus TJRA cohort. Bootstrap 95% CI using the percentile method.

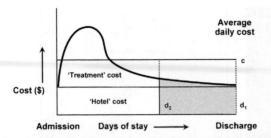

Fig. 2. Estimating the cost savings associated with reductions in hospital length-of-stay. Hospital stays include a daily fixed cost, called the *hotel cost.* Additionally, a *treatment cost* is added to each hospital day. During hospitalization, the treatment costs are often greatest during the initial portion of the hospital stay, reflecting greater care demands during a patient's initial illness. The result is that decreasing the length-of-stay from d_1 to d_2 at the end of hospitalization will likely not result in the same amount of savings as the daily average cost (*line c*) estimates. (*From* Drummond MF. Methods for the Economic Evaluation of Health Care Programmes. 3rd ed. New York: Oxford University Press. 2005; with permission.)

Finally, clinical pathways that incorporate regional anesthesia and peripheral nerve blockade may increase the likelihood of residual motor blockade, which may impede early mobilization, increase the risk of patient falls, and prolong hospital length-of-stay [43,79–82]. Kandasami and colleagues [80] recently reported a fall rate of 2% in patients undergoing total knee arthroplasty with the use of femoral nerve blockade. Fall-related injuries included wound dehiscence (n = 4) and periprosthetic fracture (n = 1). Hospital lengths-of-stay were extended 10 to 42 days secondary to complications from the fall. It has been argued, however, that residual motor blockade is a multifactorial phenomenon and cannot be entirely attributed to regional anesthesia. In addition to local anesthetic-induced quadriceps weakness, it is believed that motor block can occur secondary to surgical pain, muscle spasm, joint stiffness, swelling, dysesthesias, or other surgical factors [83]. Regardless of the cause, anesthesia providers need to play their role in minimizing the risk of residual motor blockade in patients undergoing total hip and total knee arthroplasty. Clinical pathways that incorporate peripheral nerve blockade need to do so in such a way that the benefits of regional anesthesia are achieved (ie, identifying the optimal local anesthetic, dose, and concentration), whereas the contemporary concerns of delayed rehabilitation, prolonged hospital length-of-stay, and increased hospital costs are avoided.

SUMMARY
Total hip and total knee arthroplasty are two of the most commonly performed surgical procedures in the United States with increased volumes expected over the next several decades. Clinical pathways represent a standardized, evidence-based approach to patient care designed to enhance the quality, improve the

safety, and reduce the cost associated with surgical procedures. Clinical pathways for total joint arthroplasty have been shown to significantly improve the perioperative outcomes of patients undergoing joint replacement surgery. Effective clinical pathways include preoperative patient education, a multimodal analgesic regimen, peripheral nerve blockade, standardized pain assessment and medical record documentation, pain management protocols, staff education, and early and accelerated rehabilitation. Potential clinical benefits include superior postoperative analgesia, fewer opioid-related side effects, earlier ambulation, improved joint range-of-motion, fewer postoperative complications, and reduced hospital lengths-of-stay. The financial benefits of clinical pathways include a reduction in both total hospital and direct medical costs. Further study is needed, however, to determine precisely which components of a comprehensive clinical pathway are most active in contributing to these clinical and financial benefits.

References

[1] Barbieri A, Vanhaecht K, Van Herck P, et al. Effects of clinical pathways in the joint replacement: a meta-analysis. BMC Med 2009;7:32.

[2] Panella M, Marchisio S, Di Stanislao F. Reducing clinical variations with clinical pathways: do pathways work? Int J Qual Health Care 2003;15(6):509–21.

[3] Kim S, Losina E, Solomon DH, et al. Effectiveness of clinical pathways for total knee and total hip arthroplasty: literature review. J Arthroplasty 2003;18(1):69–74.

[4] Macario A, Horne M, Goodman S, et al. The effect of a perioperative clinical pathway for knee replacement surgery on hospital costs. Anesth Analg 1998;86(5):978–84.

[5] Williams BA, Kentor ML. Clinical pathways and the anesthesiologist. Curr Anesth Reports 2000;2:418–24.

[6] Bondy LR, Sims N, Schroeder DR, et al. The effect of anesthetic patient education on preoperative patient anxiety. Reg Anesth Pain Med 1999;24(2):158–64.

[7] Lin YK, Su JY, Lin GT, et al. Impact of a clinical pathway for total knee arthroplasty. Kaohsiung J Med Sci 2002;18(3):134–40.

[8] McDonald S, Hetrick S, Green S. Pre-operative education for hip or knee replacement. Cochrane Database Syst Rev 2004;1:CD003526.

[9] Pour AE, Parvizi J, Sharkey PF, et al. Minimally invasive hip arthroplasty: what role does patient preconditioning play? J Bone Joint Surg Am 2007;89(9):1920–7.

[10] Capdevila X, Macaire P, Dadure C, et al. Continuous psoas compartment block for postoperative analgesia after total hip arthroplasty: new landmarks, technical guidelines, and clinical evaluation. Anesth Analg 2002;94(6):1606–13, table of contents.

[11] Tali M, Maaroos J. Lower limbs function and pain relationships after unilateral total knee arthroplasty. Int J Rehabil Res 2010;33(3):264–7.

[12] Horlocker TT, Kopp SL, Pagnano MW, et al. Analgesia for total hip and knee arthroplasty: a multimodal pathway featuring peripheral nerve block. J Am Acad Orthop Surg 2006;14(3):126–35.

[13] Elia N, Lysakowski C, Tramer MR. Does multimodal analgesia with acetaminophen, nonsteroidal antiinflammatory drugs, or selective cyclooxygenase-2 inhibitors and patient-controlled analgesia morphine offer advantages over morphine alone? Meta-analyses of randomized trials. Anesthesiology 2005;103(6):1296–304.

[14] Fassoulaki A, Triga A, Melemeni A, et al. Multimodal analgesia with gabapentin and local anesthetics prevents acute and chronic pain after breast surgery for cancer. Anesth Analg 2005;101(5):1427–32.

[15] Jin F, Chung F. Multimodal analgesia for postoperative pain control. J Clin Anesth 2001;13(7):524–39.

[16] Straube S, Derry S, McQuay HJ, et al. Effect of preoperative Cox-II-selective NSAIDs (cox-ibs) on postoperative outcomes: a systematic review of randomized studies. Acta Anaesthesiol Scand 2005;49(5):601–13.

[17] Maheshwari AV, Boutary M, Yun AG, et al. Multimodal analgesia without routine parenteral narcotics for total hip arthroplasty. Clin Orthop Relat Res 2006;453:231–8.

[18] Buvanendran A, Kroin JS, Tuman KJ, et al. Effects of perioperative administration of a selective cyclooxygenase 2 inhibitor on pain management and recovery of function after knee replacement: a randomized controlled trial. JAMA 2003;290(18):2411–8.

[19] Hebl JR, Kopp SL, Ali MH, et al. A comprehensive anesthesia protocol that emphasizes peripheral nerve blockade for total knee and total hip arthroplasty. J Bone Joint Surg Am 2005;87(Suppl 2):63–70.

[20] Hebl JR, Dilger JA, Byer DE, et al. A pre-emptive multimodal pathway featuring peripheral nerve block improves perioperative outcomes after major orthopedic surgery. Reg Anesth Pain Med 2008;33(6):510–7.

[21] Buvanendran A, Kroin JS, Della Valle CJ, et al. Perioperative oral pregabalin reduces chronic pain after total knee arthroplasty: a prospective, randomized, controlled trial. Anesth Analg 2010;110(1):199–207.

[22] Remerand F, Le Tendre C, Baud A, et al. The early and delayed analgesic effects of ketamine after total hip arthroplasty: a prospective, randomized, controlled, double-blind study. Anesth Analg 2009;109(6):1963–71.

[23] Fischer HB, Simanski CJ, Sharp C, et al. A procedure-specific systematic review and consensus recommendations for postoperative analgesia following total knee arthroplasty. Anaesthesia 2008;63(10):1105–23.

[24] Parvizi J, Miller AG, Gandhi K. Multimodal pain management after total joint arthroplasty. J Bone Joint Surg Am 2011;93(11):1075–84.

[25] Sinatra RS, Jahr JS, Reynolds LW, et al. Efficacy and safety of single and repeated administration of 1 gram intravenous acetaminophen injection (paracetamol) for pain management after major orthopedic surgery. Anesthesiology 2005;102(4):822–31.

[26] Silvanto M, Lappi M, Rosenberg PH. Comparison of the opioid-sparing efficacy of diclofenac and ketoprofen for 3 days after knee arthroplasty. Acta Anaesthesiol Scand 2002;46(3):322–8.

[27] Cousins MJ, Power I, Smith G. 1996 Labat lecture: pain—a persistent problem. Reg Anesth Pain Med 2000;25(1):6–21.

[28] Nikolajsen L, Brandsborg B, Lucht U, et al. Chronic pain following total hip arthroplasty: a nationwide questionnaire study. Acta Anaesthesiol Scand 2006;50(4):495–500.

[29] Brander VA, Stulberg SD, Adams AD, et al. Predicting total knee replacement pain: a prospective, observational study. Clin Orthop Relat Res 2003;(416):27–36.

[30] Perkins FM, Kehlet H. Chronic pain as an outcome of surgery. A review of predictive factors. Anesthesiology 2000;93(4):1123–33.

[31] Peters ML, Sommer M, de Rijke JM, et al. Somatic and psychologic predictors of long-term unfavorable outcome after surgical intervention. Ann Surg 2007;245(3):487–94.

[32] Allen HW, Liu SS, Ware PD, et al. Peripheral nerve blocks improve analgesia after total knee replacement surgery. Anesth Analg 1998;87(1):93–7.

[33] Wang H, Boctor B, Verner J. The effect of single-injection femoral nerve block on rehabilitation and length of hospital stay after total knee replacement. Reg Anesth Pain Med 2002;27(2):139–44.

[34] Szczukowski MJ Jr, Hines JA, Snell JA, et al. Femoral nerve block for total knee arthroplasty patients: a method to control postoperative pain. J Arthroplasty 2004;19(6):720–5.

[35] YaDeau JT, Cahill JB, Zawadsky MW, et al. The effects of femoral nerve blockade in conjunction with epidural analgesia after total knee arthroplasty. Anesth Analg 2005;101(3):891–5, table of contents.

[36] Edwards ND, Wright EM. Continuous low-dose 3-in-1 nerve blockade for postoperative pain relief after total knee replacement. Anesth Analg 1992;75(2):265–7.

[37] Singelyn FJ, Deyaert M, Joris D, et al. Effects of intravenous patient-controlled analgesia with morphine, continuous epidural analgesia, and continuous three-in-one block on postoperative pain and knee rehabilitation after unilateral total knee arthroplasty. Anesth Analg 1998;87(1):88–92.

[38] Ganapathy S, Wasserman RA, Watson JT, et al. Modified continuous femoral three-in-one block for postoperative pain after total knee arthroplasty. Anesth Analg 1999;89(5): 1197–202.

[39] Kaloul I, Guay J, Cote C, et al. The posterior lumbar plexus (psoas compartment) block and the three-in-one femoral nerve block provide similar postoperative analgesia after total knee replacement. Can J Anaesth 2004;51(1):45–51.

[40] Siddiqui ZI, Cepeda MS, Denman W, et al. Continuous lumbar plexus block provides improved analgesia with fewer side effects compared with systemic opioids after hip arthroplasty: a randomized controlled trial. Reg Anesth Pain Med 2007;32(5):393–8.

[41] Richman JM, Liu SS, Courpas G, et al. Does continuous peripheral nerve block provide superior pain control to opioids? A meta-analysis. Anesth Analg 2006;102(1):248–57.

[42] Biboulet P, Morau D, Aubas P, et al. Postoperative analgesia after total-hip arthroplasty: comparison of intravenous patient-controlled analgesia with morphine and single injection of femoral nerve or psoas compartment block a prospective, randomized, double-blind study. Reg Anesth Pain Med 2004;29(2):102–9.

[43] Ilfeld BM, Ball ST, Gearen PF, et al. Ambulatory continuous posterior lumbar plexus nerve blocks after hip arthroplasty: a dual-center, randomized, triple-masked, placebo-controlled trial. Anesthesiology 2008;109(3):491–501.

[44] Fowler SJ, Symons J, Sabato S, et al. Epidural analgesia compared with peripheral nerve blockade after major knee surgery: a systematic review and meta-analysis of randomized trials. Br J Anaesth 2008;100(2):154–64.

[45] Barrington MJ, Watts SA, Gledhill SR, et al. Preliminary results of the Australasian Regional Anaesthesia Collaboration: a prospective audit of more than 7000 peripheral nerve and plexus blocks for neurologic and other complications. Reg Anesth Pain Med 2009;34(6): 534–41.

[46] Auroy Y, Narchi P, Messiah A, et al. Serious complications related to regional anesthesia: results of a prospective survey in France. Anesthesiology 1997;87(3):479–86.

[47] Auroy Y, Benhamou D, Bargues L, et al. Major complications of regional anesthesia in France: the SOS Regional Anesthesia Hotline Service. Anesthesiology 2002;97(5): 1274–80.

[48] Jacob AK, Mantilla CB, Sviggum HP, et al. Perioperative nerve injury after total knee arthroplasty: regional anesthesia risk during a 20-year cohort study. Anesthesiology 2011;114(2): 311–7.

[49] Joint Commission. Pain Management Standards. 2001. Available at: http://www.joint commission.org/pain_management/. Accessed July 1, 2011.

[50] Benhamou D, Berti M, Brodner G, et al. Postoperative Analgesic THerapy Observational Survey (PATHOS): a practice pattern study in 7 central/southern European countries. Pain 2008;136(1–2):134–41.

[51] Fletcher D, Fermanian C, Mardaye A, et al. A patient-based national survey on postoperative pain management in France reveals significant achievements and persistent challenges. Pain 2008;137(2):441–51.

[52] Apfelbaum JL, Chen C, Mehta SS, et al. Postoperative pain experience: results from a national survey suggest postoperative pain continues to be undermanaged. Anesth Analg 2003;97(2):534–40, table of contents.

[53] Strohbuecker B, Mayer H, Evers GC, et al. Pain prevalence in hospitalized patients in a German university teaching hospital. J Pain Symptom Manage 2005;29(5):498–506.

[54] Harmer M, Davies KA. The effect of education, assessment and a standardised prescription on postoperative pain management. The value of clinical audit in the establishment of acute pain services. Anaesthesia 1998;53(5):424–30.

[55] Munin MC, Rudy TE, Glynn NW, et al. Early inpatient rehabilitation after elective hip and knee arthroplasty. JAMA 1998;279(11):847–52.

[56] Mahomed NN, Davis AM, Hawker G, et al. Inpatient compared with home-based rehabilitation following primary unilateral total hip or knee replacement: a randomized controlled trial. J Bone Joint Surg Am 2008;90(8):1673–80.

[57] Skinner HB, Shintani EY. Results of a multimodal analgesic trial involving patients with total hip or total knee arthroplasty. Am J Orthop (Belle Mead NJ) 2004;33(2):85–92 [discussion: 92].

[58] Peters CL, Shirley B, Erickson J. The effect of a new multimodal perioperative anesthetic regimen on postoperative pain, side effects, rehabilitation, and length of hospital stay after total joint arthroplasty. J Arthroplasty 2006;21(6 Suppl 2):132–8.

[59] Salinas FV, Liu SS, Mulroy MF. The effect of single-injection femoral nerve block versus continuous femoral nerve block after total knee arthroplasty on hospital length-of-stay and long-term functional recovery within an established clinical pathway. Anesth Analg 2006;102(4):1234–9.

[60] DeFrances CJ, Podgornik MN. 2004 National Hospital Discharge Survey. Adv Data 2006;(371):1–19.

[61] Bozic KJ, Beringer D. Economic considerations in minimally invasive total joint arthroplasty. Clin Orthop Relat Res 2007;463:20–5.

[62] Duncan CM, Hall Long K, Warner DO, et al. The economic implications of a multimodal analgesic regimen for patients undergoing major orthopedic surgery: a comparative study of direct costs. Reg Anesth Pain Med 2009;34(4):301–7.

[63] Quality AfHra. HCUPnet Healthcare Cost and Utilization Project. Rockville (MD): Agency for Healthcare Research and Quality; 2004.

[64] Kurtz S, Ong K, Lau E, et al. Projections of primary and revision hip and knee arthroplasty in the United States from 2005 to 2030. J Bone Joint Surg Am 2007;89(4):780–5.

[65] Singh JA, Vessely MB, Harmsen WS, et al. A population-based study of trends in the use of total hip and total knee arthroplasty, 1969-2008. Mayo Clin Proc 2010;85(10): 898–904.

[66] Ong KL, Mowat FS, Chan N, et al. Economic burden of revision hip and knee arthroplasty in Medicare enrollees. Clin Orthop Relat Res 2006;446:22–8.

[67] ISPOR. Health care cost, quality and outcomes. ISPOR Book of Terms. Lawrenceville (NJ): International Society for Pharmacoeconomics and Outcomes Research; 2003.

[68] Fisher DA, Trimble S, Clapp B, et al. Effect of a patient management system on outcomes of total hip and knee arthroplasty. Clin Orthop Relat Res 1997;(345):155–60.

[69] Healy WL, Iorio R, Ko J, et al. Impact of cost reduction programs on short-term patient outcome and hospital cost of total knee arthroplasty. J Bone Joint Surg Am 2002;84(3): 348–53.

[70] Lucas CE, Vlahos AL, Ledgerwood AM. Kindness kills: the negative impact of pain as the fifth vital sign. J Am Coll Surg 2007;205(1):101–7.

[71] Mabrey JD, Toohey JS, Armstrong DA, et al. Clinical pathway management of total knee arthroplasty. Clin Orthop Relat Res 1997;(345):125–33.

[72] Wammack L, Mabrey JD. Outcomes assessment of total hip and total knee arthroplasty: critical pathways, variance analysis, and continuous quality improvement. Clin Nurse Spec 1998;12(3):122–9 [quiz: 130–1].

[73] Brunenberg DE, van Steyn MJ, Sluimer JC, et al. Joint recovery programme versus usual care: an economic evaluation of a clinical pathway for joint replacement surgery. Med Care 2005;43(10):1018–26.

[74] Ireson CL. Critical pathways: effectiveness in achieving patient outcomes. J Nurs Adm 1997;27(6):16–23.

[75] Drummond MF. Methods for the economic evaluation of health care programmes. 3rd edition. Oxford (NY): Oxford University Press; 2005.

[76] Taylor S, Voytovich AE, Kozol RA. Has the pendulum swung too far in postoperative pain control? Am J Surg 2003;186(5):472–5.

[77] Taylor S, Kirton OC, Staff I, et al. Postoperative day one: a high risk period for respiratory events. Am J Surg 2005;190(5):752–6.

[78] Vila H Jr, Smith RA, Augustyniak MJ, et al. The efficacy and safety of pain management before and after implementation of hospital-wide pain management standards: is patient safety compromised by treatment based solely on numerical pain ratings? Anesth Analg 2005;101(2):474–80, table of contents.

[79] Ilfeld BM, Le LT, Meyer RS, et al. Ambulatory continuous femoral nerve blocks decrease time to discharge readiness after tricompartment total knee arthroplasty: a randomized, triple-masked, placebo-controlled study. Anesthesiology 2008;108(4):703–13.

[80] Kandasami M, Kinninmonth AW, Sarungi M, et al. Femoral nerve block for total knee replacement—a word of caution. Knee 2009;16(2):98–100.

[81] Klein SM, Nielsen KC, Greengrass RA, et al. Ambulatory discharge after long-acting peripheral nerve blockade: 2382 blocks with ropivacaine. Anesth Analg 2002;94(1):65–70, table of contents.

[82] Williams BA, Kentor ML, Bottegal MT. The incidence of falls at home in patients with perineural femoral catheters: a retrospective summary of a randomized clinical trial. Anesth Analg 2007;104(4):1002.

[83] Barrington MJ, Olive D, Low K, et al. Continuous femoral nerve blockade or epidural analgesia after total knee replacement: a prospective randomized controlled trial. Anesth Analg 2005;101(6):1824–9.

ADVANCES IN ANESTHESIA

INDEX

Note: Page numbers of article titles are in **boldface** type.

0737-6146/11/$ – see front matter
doi:10.1016/S0737-6146(11)00018-9

Printed and bound by CPI Group (UK) Ltd, Croydon, CR0 4YY

08/05/2025

01864677-0020